Grammar & Writing Skills for the
Health Professional

Grammar & Writing Skills for the Health Professional

Third Edition

Doreen Villemaire Oberg

M.Ed., RN, CMA

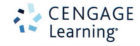

CENGAGE
Learning®

Australia • Brazil • Mexico • Singapore • United Kingdom • United States

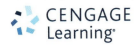

Grammar and Writing Skills for the Health Professional, Third Edition

Doreen Villemaire Oberg

SVP, GM Skills & Global Product Management: Dawn Gerrain

Product Director: Matthew Seeley

Product Manager: Laura Stewart

Senior Director, Development: Marah Bellegarde

Senior Product Development Manager: Juliet Steiner

Senior Content Developer: Darcy M. Scelsi

Product Assistant: Deborah Handy

Vice President, Marketing Services: Jennifer Ann Baker

Marketing Manager: Jessica Cipperly

Senior Production Director: Wendy Troeger

Production Director: Andrew Crouth

Senior Content Project Manager: Kenneth McGrath

Senior Art Director: Jack Pendleton

Cover image(s): iStock.com/Cesair; iStock .com/Steve Debenport; Stock.com /RuslanDashinsky; iStock.com/ilyast; iStock.com/Yuzach

For product information and technology assistance, contact us at **Cengage Learning Customer & Sales Support, 1-800-354-9706**

For permission to use material from this text or product, submit all requests online at **www.cengage.com/permissions** Further permissions questions can be e-mailed to **permissionrequest@cengage.com**

Library of Congress Control Number: 2016948336

ISBN: 978-1-3059-4542-5

Cengage Learning
20 Channel Center Street
Boston, MA 02210
USA

Cengage Learning is a leading provider of customized learning solutions with employees residing in nearly 40 different countries and sales in more than 125 countries around the world. Find your local representative at **www.cengage.com**

Cengage Learning products are represented in Canada by Nelson Education, Ltd.

To learn more about Cengage Learning, visit **www.cengage.com**

Purchase any of our products at your local college store or at our preferred online store **www.cengagebrain.com**

Notice to the Reader

Publisher does not warrant or guarantee any of the products described herein or perform any independent analysis in connection with any of the product information contained herein. Publisher does not assume, and expressly disclaims, any obligation to obtain and include information other than that provided to it by the manufacturer. The reader is expressly warned to consider and adopt all safety precautions that might be indicated by the activities described herein and to avoid all potential hazards. By following the instructions contained herein, the reader willingly assumes all risks in connection with such instructions. The publisher makes no representations or warranties of any kind, including but not limited to, the warranties of fitness for particular purpose or merchantability, nor are any such representations implied with respect to the material set forth herein, and the publisher takes no responsibility with respect to such material. The publisher shall not be liable for any special, consequential, or exemplary damages resulting, in whole or part, from the readers' use of, or reliance upon, this material.

Printed in the United States of America
Print Number: 01   Print Year: 2016

Contents

MODULE 1: The Basics of Grammar

SECTION 1: Nouns 3

Objectives   3
Introduction   3
Nouns   4
  Proper and Common Nouns   4
  Collective Nouns   5
  Concrete Nouns   6
  Abstract Nouns   6
Noun Plurals   7
  Forming Plurals of Nouns in General   7
  Forming the Plurals of Medical Terms   7
Functions of Nouns   9
  Nominative Case: Subject   10
  Nominative Case: Predicate Noun   10

Objective Case   11
Possessive Case   12
Appositives and Direct Address   14
Nouns Summary   15
Medical Spelling   17
Real-World Applications   17
  Medical Office Correspondence   17
    The Medical Letter   17
    Letter Components   18
  Addressing Envelopes   28
    Folding the Letter   29
Skills Review   29
Comprehensive Review   32

SECTION 2: Pronouns 35

Objectives   35
Introduction   35

Pronouns   36
  Personal Pronouns   36

Gender   36
Number and Person   36
Nominative Case (Subject)   37
Nominative Case (Predicate)   38
Objective Case   39
Possessive Case   39
Reflexive Pronouns   40
Relative Pronouns   41
Indefinite Pronouns   42
Interrogative Pronouns   43
Demonstrative Pronouns   44
Pronoun-Antecedent Agreement   45

Number   45
Gender   45
Pronoun Summary   47
Medical Spelling   48
Real-World Applications   48
The Office Memorandum and Electronic Mail   48
Writing a Memo or an Email   48
Office Memorandum and Electronic Mail Summary   52
Skills Review   53
Comprehensive Review   55

SECTION 3: Verbs 57

Objectives   57
Verbs   57
Action Verbs   57
"Being" Verbs   58
Main Verbs and Helping Verbs   59
Linking Verbs   59
Transitive and Intransitive Verbs   60
Gerunds   61
Infinitives   61
Person of a Verb   61
Number of a Verb   62
Verb Tenses   63
Present Tense   63
Past Tense   63
Future Tense   64
Principal Parts of Verbs   65
Regular Verbs   65
Irregular Verbs   66
Confusing and Troublesome Verbs   69

Lie and Lay   69
Rise and Raise   69
May and Can   70
Use of Verb Tenses in Sentences   71
Voices of Verbs   72
Active and Passive Verbs   72
The Passive Voice   73
Moods of Verbs   74
Verbs Summary   75
Medical Spelling   76
Real-World Applications   76
The Medical Record   76
The American Health Information Management Association   77
Joint Commission   77
The Health Insurance Portability and Accountability Act of 1996   79
Skills Review   81
Comprehensive Review   84

SECTION 4: Adjectives 87

Objectives   87
Adjectives   87
Limiting Adjectives   88
A and AN   88
Singular and Plural   89
Interrogative and Proper Adjectives   90
Predicate and Compound Adjectives   90
Descriptive Adjectives   92
Placement of Adjectives   94

Modifiers and Placement   94
Degrees of Adjectives to Express Comparison   96
Positive   96
Comparative   96
Superlative   97
Other Comparisons   98
Troublesome Adjectives   99
Eponyms   100

Adjectives Summary   100
Medical Spelling   101
Real-World Applications   101
   Medical Reports   101
   Radiology and Imaging Report   102
   Pathology Report   103

Discharge Summary   104
   Operative Report   104
Medical Reports Summary   106
Skills Review   107
Comprehensive Review   110

SECTION 5: Adverbs *113*

Objectives   113
Adverbs   113
Adverbs as Modifiers   115
Frequency of Adverbs   116
Degrees of Comparison   116
   Positive   116
   Comparative   116
   Superlative   117
   Irregular Adverbs   117
      Using Most and More   *117*
Changing Adjectives into Adverbs   118
Negative Adverbs   119
   "Not" as a Contraction   119
   Double Negatives   120

Placement of Adverbs   121
Troublesome Adverbs   121
Adverbs Summary   122
Medical Spelling   122
Real-World Applications   123
   Fax, Phone Courtesy, Messages,
   and Minutes of a Meeting   123
      Facsimile   *123*
      Telephone Courtesy and Messages   *123*
      Minutes of a Meeting   *125*
Fax, Phone Message, and Minutes
   of a Meeting Summary   127
Skills Review   128
Comprehensive Review   130

MODULE 2: Advanced Grammar

SECTION 6: The Sentence *135*

Objectives   135
Introduction   135
Components of the Sentence   136
   Independent and Dependent Clause   136
      Types of Dependent Clauses   *137*
   Phrases   138
      Prepositional Phrases   *139*
      Participial Phrase   *139*
      Gerund Phrase   *140*
      Infinitive Phrase   *140*
Sentence Structure   141
   Simple Sentences   141
   Compound Sentences   141
   Complex Sentences   142
   Compound-Complex Sentences   142
Classifications of Sentences   143

Declarative Sentences   143
Imperative Sentences   143
Interrogative Sentences   143
Exclamatory Sentences   144
Effective Sentences   144
   Parallel Structure   145
   Conciseness   146
   Diction   149
   Positive Statements   151
Ineffective Sentences   152
   The Fragmented Sentence   152
   The Comma Splice   153
   The Run-On Sentence   153
Sentence Summary   154
Phrases Summary   155
Medical Spelling   157

Real-World Applications 157
   Progress Notes, Charting, and
   Documenting 157
      Traditional Charting 158
      SOAP 158
      SOAPE 160

SOAPIE 160
SOAPIER 160
PIE 160
Charting and Documenting Summary 161
Skills Review 162
Comprehensive Review 163

SECTION 7: Punctuation 167

Objectives 167
Punctuation 167
   The Period 168
   The Question Mark 169
   The Exclamation Point 169
   The Comma 170
   The Semicolon 173
   The Colon 175
   Parentheses 176
   The Dash 177
   The Hyphen 177
   The Apostrophe 178

Italics 179
   Quotation Marks 180
Punctuation Summary 181
Medical Spelling 183
Real-World Applications 183
   Medical Reports 183
      History and Physical Reports 183
      Consultation Report 185
Medical Reports Summary 185
Skills Review 187
Comprehensive Review 188

SECTION 8: Prepositions, Conjunctions, and Paragraphs 191

Objectives 191
Prepositions 191
   Compound Prepositions 193
   Prepositional Phrases 195
      Prepositional Noun/Pronoun
      Modifiers 195
      Prepositional Verb Modifiers 196
   Problematic Prepositions 197
   Prepositions at the End of a Sentence 199
Conjunctions 200
   Coordinating Conjunctions 200
   Correlative Conjunctions 200
   Subordinating Conjunctions 201
Prepositions and Conjunctions
   Summary 201
Medical Spelling 203
Paragraphs 203
   Types of Paragraphs 205
      Narrative Paragraph 205
      Descriptive Paragraph 205

Expository Paragraph 206
Persuasive Paragraph 206
Structure of a Paragraph 207
   Topic Sentence 207
   Supporting Sentences 207
   Concluding Sentence 207
Putting the Paragraph Together 208
Paragraph Organization 209
Paragraph Unity 212
Paragraph Summary 213
Medical Spelling 214
Real-World Applications 214
   Medical Writing 214
      Manuscripts and Research 214
      Promotional Writing 215
Research, Manuscripts, and Promotional
   Writing Summary 218
Skills Review 219
Comprehensive Review 223

MODULE 3: Putting It All Together

SECTION 9: The Writing Process 227

Objectives   227
Introduction   227
The Writing Process   228
  Step One: Prewriting   228
  Step Two: Writing   228
  Step Three: Rewriting   229
  Step Four: Finalizing   230

Step Five: Proofreading   230
Writing Style   231
Computer Writing   234
Guidelines for Effective Writing Summary   235
Medical Spelling   235
Skills Review   236
Comprehensive Review   238

SECTION 10: The Resume and Cover Letter 241

Objectives   241
The Resume   241
  Essentials of the Resume   241
  Your Objective   242
  The Importance of Keywords   242
  Types of Resumes   243
  Wrapping It Up   245
The Cover Letter   246
Skills Review   248
Comprehensive Review   248

Appendices
  Appendix A: Spelling Rules   251
  Appendix B: Capitalization Rules   255
  Appendix C: Number Use   257
  Appendix D: Clichés   259
  Appendix E: Titles and Salutations   261
  Appendix F: Use of a Thesaurus   266
  Appendix G: Use of the English Dictionary   267
  Appendix H: Use of the Medical Dictionary   270

Glossary   271
Index   277

Preface

Dear Students:

Welcome to the medical world! The words may be a little different. This message is for you. This book will offer you the advantage of learning the grammar, some medical words, and introduce some writings of the profession you are entering during any part of your curriculum. It is meant to give an entry level student in the health care profession some guidelines and practical knowledge in the grammar and writing world. It is an introduction to the skills and tools that will be needed for your new job ahead.

The world is moving in a very fast technological direction. Computers and technology have rapidly influenced our human culture. It isn't just about handheld calculators anymore, but also smartphones, tablets, laptops, and more technology still to come. We need to learn and add the knowledge of software and computers to everything in life.

Writing can be done anywhere. As recently as a few generations ago it was important to find a place away from the hustle and bustle of life—perhaps a room, a library, or a desk area—where one could work and think; today it is about finding a comfortable place—any place—where one can tune in to connect and learn. Learn to be in your own space for thinking and learning and producing new, wonderful thoughts.

Many health care professionals have several different duties that require a variety of skills. A few examples of typical duties and skills of the Medical Assistant are: Answering the phones and assessing the patient's need for an appointment, taking vital signs, administering medications, assisting in minor surgeries, administering electrocardiogram, scheduling appointments, processing insurance claims, giving injections, scheduling diagnostic tests, working with the medical record, and medical coding and billing. A few very important points as you begin:

1. Understand that being submerged in the private world of patient confidentiality is extremely important. It is vital that the medical professional keeps the confidentiality, dignity, and privacy of patients. With the new laws and legal issues that have evolved along with HIPAA, which we discuss later, it is imperative that employees do not discuss patients verbally or on the computer with anyone other than the patient's physician.

2. Remember to smile, be kind, and keep a positive attitude. I leave you with the following advice:

"Attitude" by Charles R. Swindoll

"The longer I live, the more I realize the impact of attitude on life. Attitude, to me, is more important than facts. It is more important than the past, than education, than money, than circumstances, than failures, than successes, than what other people think or say or do. It is more important than appearance, giftedness or skill. It will make or break a company ... a church ... a home. The remarkable thing is we have a choice everyday regarding the attitude we embrace for that day. We cannot change our past ... we cannot change the fact that people will act in a certain way ... We cannot change the inevitable. The only thing we can do is play on the one string we have, and that is **our attitude**. I am convinced that life is 10% what happens to me and 90% of how I react to it. And so it is with you ... we are in charge of our attitudes."

I wish you the very best as you embark on this journey.

Dear Instructors:
It is my desire to help the people who want to work in the medical/health professions to learn the words and writings, or the reports and documenting of the health field. Teaching has changed dramatically over the years, especially since many students now use English as a second language. In this busy world there is less time for the little things that may someday become a major factor in one's professional life.

This text has changed to help you, the instructor, as well as the students.

My journey with Cengage Learning has brought the arrangement of the text in this way:

- The book is divided into three modules and ten sections that can be interchanged throughout a curriculum or the sections can be used separately. There are practices, practical applications, and reviews for the student at the end of every section. Employers do prefer to hire medical assistants and medical health professionals that have received formal training and know the essentials of grammar and writing.

- The book has been arranged for its usefulness. It can be used alone as a "Grammar and Writing Class for the Health Professional" or incorporated into other classes as a supplemental book or adjunct.

- Module 1 contains five sections and covers the basics of grammar, the knowledge that is needed to communicate effectively.

- Module 2 contains three sections and covers the building and linking of all the basic grammar into sentences. This module brings punctuation and paragraphs into the center of grammar and writing for the medical assistant. The instructor may choose to use part of one section or include all sections.

- Module 3 contains two sections and covers learning to write using "The Writing Process" and putting the information from the lessons together. It includes a new section on Resumes.

I wish you the very best and I hope you find this text useful and rewarding.

Blessings,
Doreen Villemaire Oberg

New to This Edition

The new edition has been divided into Modules with multiple sections per module. Writing process worksheets have been removed from each chapter.

Module 1: Basics of Grammar—Covers nouns, pronouns, verbs, adjectives, and adverbs.

Section 1

- Formerly Chapter 2
- Omitted discussion of gender nouns
- Reduced the content on folding letters

Section 2

- Formerly Chapter 3

Section 3

- Formerly Chapter 4
- Added discussion of AHIM and Joint Commission
- Updated and expanded discussion of HIPAA

Section 4

- Formerly Chapter 7

Section 5

- Formerly Chapter 8

Module 2: Advanced Grammar—Consists of sentence structure, punctuation, and prepositions.

Section 6

- Formerly Chapter 5 and Chapter 10—These have now been combined.
- Promotional Writing was moved to Section 8.

Section 7

- Formerly Chapter 6

Section 8

- Formerly Chapter 9 and Chapter 11—These have now been combined.
- Condensed content on Medical Writing

Module 3: Putting It All Together—Focuses on the writing process and resume writing

Section 9

- Formerly Chapter 1

Section 10

- New chapter on writing resumes and cover letters

MODULE 1

The Basics of Grammar

SECTION 1
Nouns

Practical Writing Component: Medical Correspondence and Letters

Objectives

After reading this section, the learner should be able to:

- identify basic types of nouns.
- identify nouns by number and function.
- explain the difference between apposition and direct address.
- spell various medical terms.
- form the plurals of regular nouns and medical nouns.
- prepare medical letters with accompanying envelope.
- identify medical nouns.

 # Introduction

Grammar is a set of rules about words and how they are used in sentences for the purpose of conveying a message. A sentence is a group of words that expresses a complete thought. The individual words that make up a sentence are called *parts of speech* (Figure 1-1). The parts of speech are:

Noun	names a person, place, thing, or idea
Pronoun	substitutes for a noun
Verb	shows action, being, or linking
Adjective	describes a noun or pronoun
Adverb	describes a verb, adjective, or other adverb
Preposition	shows relationship to a noun or pronoun
Conjunction	connects words or groups of words
Article	points out or limits

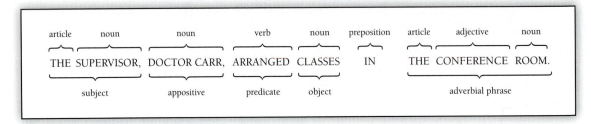

FIGURE 1-1 Sentence Structure

"Parts of speech" direct the manner in which words are used in sentences. Good language skills are critical to any professional success. It is a continuous learning cycle. Honing language skills will increase comprehension in all classes.

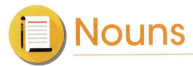

Nouns

Nouns are used more frequently than any other part of speech. Sentences abound with them. Every sentence you read, write, speak, hear, text, or email contains nouns. Note the number of nouns (in italic) in this sentence:

The *supervisor, Doctor Carr,* arranged *classes* in the conference *room*.

A *noun* is a word used to name a person, place, object (thing, activity), or quality (idea). The types of nouns covered in this chapter are proper, common, collective, concrete, and abstract.

Proper and Common Nouns

Proper and common nouns are easy to understand. A *proper noun* names a particular person, place, object, or quality. To help remember the definition, think of the words *proper* and *particular* that both begin with the letter *P*. Words like *Main Street, Dr. Villes, Massachusetts, Memorial Hospital, American Association of Medical Assistants (A.A.M.A.), Red Cross,* and *University Hospital* are proper nouns. Proper nouns begin with a capital letter.

Common nouns do not name any specific or particular person, place, object, or quality. They are general words such as *book, vegetable, hospital, patient, artery, muscle, temperature, admission, bacteria, examination, physician, specimen,* and *bone*. Common nouns do not begin with a capital letter.

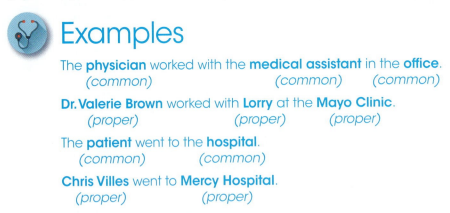

Examples

The **physician** worked with the **medical assistant** in the **office**.
(common)   *(common)*   *(common)*

Dr. Valerie Brown worked with **Lorry** at the **Mayo Clinic**.
(proper)   *(proper)*   *(proper)*

The **patient** went to the **hospital**.
(common)   *(common)*

Chris Villes went to **Mercy Hospital**.
(proper)   *(proper)*

Eponyms are often encountered in the medical field and these are proper nouns. Eponyms are sur- names of people used as descriptive adjectives for diseases, instruments, syndromes, procedures, drugs, parts of the human body, and other medical nouns. Words such as *Bell's palsy, Babinski's reflex, Foley catheter,* and *Buck's extension* are eponyms. The eponym is capitalized, but not the noun following it. It is important to check the spelling of eponyms in a medical dictionary.

The names of specific departments in a hospital or clinic are capitalized proper nouns. The reference to a general department is not a proper noun and so is not capitalized.

The brand or trade name of a drug is a capitalized proper noun, but the generic or common name of the drug is not; for example, aspirin or Bayer® aspirin, and meperidine or Demerol®. When in doubt about capitalizing, consult the PDR *(Physicians' Desk Reference).*

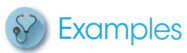 # Examples

Proper	Common
Taber's Cyclopedic Medical Dictionary	chickenpox
German measles	flu
Medical Records Department	operating room
Amoxicillin	penicillin
Tylenol	acetaminophen
Meckel's diverticulum	diverticulitis
Marshall-Marchetti operation	laparotomy

 ## PRACTICE 1: Nouns

Identify the italicized words as proper or common nouns:

1. The largest *artery* in the body is the *aorta.* _____

2. *Scientists* were watching changes in the *DNA.* _____

3. Pulmonary *veins* are the only *veins* in the *body* that carry oxygenated *blood.*

   _____

4. *Croup* is the narrowing of the air passage in the *larynx.* _____

5. *Cholesterol* is a lipid found in saturated *fats.* _____

Collective Nouns

Collective nouns are nouns that represent a group. Examples of collective nouns are:

audience	committee	faculty	nation	school
board	company	family	navy	society
choir	crew	group	panel	staff
club	crowd	jury	public	union

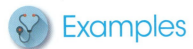

Examples

The *staff* of physicians works as a *team*.

The *family* consented to the operation.

PRACTICE 2: Nouns

Identify the collective nouns in the following sentences:

1. The patient was on the faculty at the medical school. _____

2. A group of muscles helps the movement of the mouth. _____

3. Chris joined the faculty after graduation. _____

4. The family is the basic structure of society. _____

5. The hospital welcomed the inclusion of a union. _____

Concrete Nouns

Concrete nouns are easy to identify because they name things that are touchable, visible, and audible; that is, they are perceived by the senses.

Examples

Bones and *muscles* work together.

Muscles are attached to *bones* by *tendons*.

Massachusetts General Hospital is in *Boston*.

The *New England Journal of Medicine* is an excellent *journal*.

Abstract Nouns

Abstract nouns are more difficult to identify because they name a concept, quality, or idea. Think of abstract nouns as untouchables. Abstract nouns often have *-ness, -dom, -th, -ance, -cy,* and *-ism* for endings. Examples of abstract nouns are:

acceptance	courage	foolishness	intelligence	security
accuracy	danger	freedom	love	strength
case	emotion	function	memory	theories
concept	energy	grief	method	truth
condition	evidence	honesty	personality	type

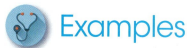

Examples

The concept portrayed the personality and honesty of the individual.

The strength of this concept lies in the facts about the musculoskeletal system.

Patience is an admirable quality in any medical assistant.

Wordiness is inexcusable in written communication.

PRACTICE 3: Nouns

State whether the italicized words are collective or abstract:

1. The Patient's Bill of Rights provides greater *satisfaction* and *care* for the patient.
   _____

2. The medical *staff* is meeting at 10 A.M. _____

3. After class, the *group* celebrated its hard work. _____

4. Members of the A.M.A. worked as a *team*. _____

5. The *evidence* is questionable. _____

Noun Plurals

When referring to more than one person, place, or thing you are using plural nouns.

Forming Plurals of Nouns in General

A few basic rules help to form the plurals of nouns (Figure 1-2). However, like many rules, there are some exceptions. When in doubt about the spelling of any word, always consult a dictionary.

Forming the Plurals of Medical Terms

Many medical terms are derived from Greek and Latin words. Forming the plurals of medical terms is somewhat different from forming the plurals of regular nouns. (Figure 1-3). Reviewing the following rules may be helpful when charting, correcting, typing, or corresponding.

1. Most singular nouns are made plural just by adding *s*: *patient, patients; bone, bones; tendon, tendons; symptom, symptoms; friend, friends; nurse, nurses; writing, writings.*

2. To form the plurals of nouns ending in *s, x, ch, sh,* and *z,* add *es*: *dress, dresses; church, churches; tax, taxes; wish, wishes; quiz, quizzes; process, processes; larynx, larynxes.*

3. Singular nouns ending in *y* preceded by a vowel form their plurals by adding *s*: *attorney, attorneys; boy, boys; x-ray, x-rays; key, keys.*

4. Nouns ending in *y* preceded by a consonant form the plural by changing *y* to *i* and adding *es*: *policy, policies; copy, copies; allergy, allergies; extremity, extremities; study, studies; dichotomy, dichotomies; deficiency, deficiencies.*

5. Singular nouns ending in *f* and *fe* form the plural in two ways. If the final *f* in the plural form is heard, add *s*: *belief, beliefs; safe, safes; staff, staffs.* If the final *f* in the plural has a *v* sound, change the *f* to *v* and add *es*: *life, lives; half, halves; wife, wives; leaf, leaves.*

6. Singular nouns ending in *o* preceded by a vowel form their plurals by adding *s*: *studio, studios; duo, duos; portfolio, portfolios.* Singular nouns ending in *o* preceded by a consonant form the plural by adding *s* or *es*: *echo, echoes; hero, heroes; two, twos; potato, potatoes.* Usage varies, so consult a dictionary when in doubt. Note that there are two acceptable plurals of *zero* (*zeros, zeroes*) and *no* (*nos, noes*).

FIGURE 1-2 Rules for Forming Plurals

1. Change *x* to *c* or *g* and add *es*: *apex, apices; thorax, thoraces; meninx, meninges; appendix, appendices; phalanx, phalanges.*

2. Change *is* to *es*: *diagnosis, diagnoses; prognosis, prognoses.*

3. Change *oma* to *omata*: *stoma, stomata; sarcoma, sarcomata; carcinoma, carcinomata* (but *carcinomas* is also acceptable).

4. Change *a* to *ae*: *sequela, sequelae; vertebra, vertebrae; pleura, pleurae.*

5. Change *um* to *a*: *ovum, ova; bacterium, bacteria; diverticulum, diverticula.*

6. Change *us* to *i*: *fungus, fungi; streptococcus, streptococci; thrombus, thrombi; bronchus, bronchi.*

7. Change *on* to *a*: *ganglion, ganglia.*

8. Change *en* to *ina*: *lumen, lumina.*

FIGURE 1-3 Rules for Forming Plurals of Medical Nouns

PRACTICE 4: Nouns

Form the plurals of the words in italics:

1. Protect *child* from electrical shock by covering unused *outlet*. _____

2. Maslow arranges human *need* into five *category*. _____

3. The *diagnosis* were negative. _____

4. Congenital *anomaly* are physical *abnormality* at birth. _____

5. There are seven cervical *vertebra*. _____

Identify the singular form of these nouns:

1. Nuclei   nuclae, nuclons, nucleus _____

2. Foci   focus, focis, focae _____

3. strata   stratae, strati, stratum _____

4. emboli   emblae, embolum, embolus _____

5. ova   ovae, ovum, ovi _____

Identify the plural form of these nouns:

1. septum   septae, section, septa _____

2. fimbria   fimbrium, fimbri, fimbriae _____

3. thorax   throaxses, thoraxae, thoraces _____

4. bronchus   bronchae, bronchi, bronchum _____

5. aponeurosis   aponeursum, aponeurosae, aponeuroses _____

Functions of Nouns

Nouns can be used in different ways in a sentence (Figure 1-4):

Subject	the person, place, thing, or idea that the sentence is about
Predicate Noun	a word that follows a *linking* verb and that tells something about the subject
Direct Object	the person, place, thing, or idea that receives the action of the verb
Indirect Object	a word that answers "to whom?" or "to what?" about the verb
Possessive Noun	a word that indicates possession or ownership by its form
Appositive	a word or group of words following a word to identify or give information about that word
Direct Address	a word or group of words naming or denoting the person or persons spoken to

The use of a noun in a sentence is described by its case, which shows its relationship to other words in the sentence. In English there are three cases: nominative (or subject), objective, and possessive (or genitive).

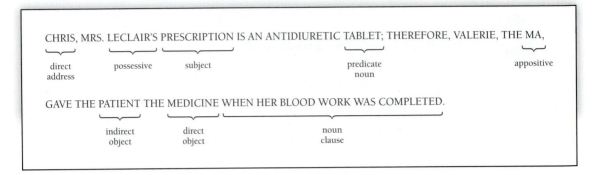

CHRIS, MRS. LECLAIR'S PRESCRIPTION IS AN ANTIDIURETIC TABLET; THEREFORE, VALERIE, THE MA,

direct   possessive   subject   predicate   appositive
address   noun

GAVE THE PATIENT THE MEDICINE WHEN HER BLOOD WORK WAS COMPLETED.

indirect   direct   noun
object   object   clause

FIGURE 1-4 Some Uses of Nouns

Nominative Case: Subject

Nominative case refers to the *subject* (abbreviated S) of a sentence. The subject is always a noun or a group of words that functions as a noun. The *subject* of a sentence is the person, place, thing, or idea about which something is said. It is determined by asking "who?" or "what?" about the verb and can be found anywhere in the sentence.

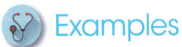 ## Examples

The *supervisor* scheduled six nurses. [Who scheduled? The *supervisor* scheduled.]

Students increased their skills with practice. [Who increased? *Students* increased.]

Bones of the skull protect the brain. [What protects? *Bones* protect.]

 ## PRACTICE 5: Nouns

Identify the subject in each sentence by placing an S above it:

1. The instructor's approach to writing excited the students.
2. The embolus traveled to the lungs.
3. The symptoms are fever and headache.
4. The ability to proofread is a plus in the doctor's office.
5. The otologist diagnosed otitis media.

Nominative Case: Predicate Noun

A noun that follows a linking verb and functions as another name for the subject is sometimes referred to as the *predicate noun*. Common *linking verbs* include: am, is, are, was, were, be, being, been. It is the same person, place, thing, or idea as the subject.

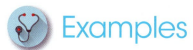

Examples

Doctors are *specialists*. [*Specialists* is a predicate noun of the subject, *Doctors; are* is the linking verb.]

Valerie is a good *friend*. [*Friend* is the predicate noun of the subject, *Valerie; is* is the linking verb.]

PRACTICE 6: Nouns

Identify the predicate noun in each sentence by placing PN above it:

1. Clothing is a nonverbal message.
2. Communication with patients is an essential skill.
3. Meninges is the term for the protective covering of the brain.
4. The patient's response to the illness was denial.
5. The elderly patient is Mrs. Leclair, the CVA in room 513.

Objective Case

The *direct object* (objective case) is a noun that follows a verb and names the person, place, thing, or idea that receives the action.

Examples

The physician dictated the *report*. (dictated what? *report*)

Can you help *Jim*? (help whom? *Jim*)

The *indirect object* is a noun that follows a verb that names the person, place, or thing **to whom, for whom, to what,** or **for what** something was done.

Examples

The patient wrote the *pharmacist* a check. (wrote to whom? *pharmacist*)

Villes Medical Associates pays its *employees* competitive salaries. (pays to whom? *employees*.)

The *object of a preposition* is a noun that follows a preposition. Some common prepositions are: *to, for, on, with, off, in, during, by,* and *over*

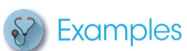

Examples

The doctor wrote a letter to the cardiologist. (*cardiologist* is the object of the preposition *to*)

Arthroscopy is visualization *with* an *endoscope*. (endoscope is the object of the preposition *with*)

PRACTICE 7: Nouns

Identify the direct object in each sentence by placing DO above it:

1. The neurologist prescribed medication for the condition.
2. The gastroenterologist did the colonoscopy.
3. Patients have a right to information in the medical record.
4. The doctor owns the medical record.
5. The cell contains complex structures.

Identify the indirect object in each sentence by placing IO above it:

1. The surgeon gave the residents an opportunity to operate.
2. The patient mailed the doctor the check.
3. The scrub nurse handed the doctor a scalpel.
4. Matthew told the Medicare class his ideas.
5. The nurse fed the patient some soup.

Identify the object of the preposition in each sentence by placing OP above it:

1. The ileum is the distal portion of the small intestines.
2. Ethics is a branch of moral science.
3. TRICARE is insurance for military families.
4. A statute of limitations fixes the period of time for legal action.
5. Skills in verbal communication are required of the health care team.

Possessive Case

Possessive case indicates possession or ownership. For example, *patient's medication* shows that the patient is the owner of the medication. *Medication* is the noun that follows the possessive noun, *patient's*. To check the accuracy of the possessive, change the words to *the medication of the patient*.

Use an apostrophe (') to form the possessive. The six rules for forming a possessive noun are listed in Figure 1-5.

1. To form the possessive of singular nouns, add an apostrophe and the letter *s* ('s) to the noun. The word that has the apostrophe is the word that owns something.

   patient's bed [the bed of the patient]

   doctor's white coat [the white coat of the doctor]

2. The possessive of plural nouns ending in *s* is formed by adding only an apostrophe after the *s* (s').

   doctors' dressing room [the dressing room of the doctors]

   nurses' scrub gowns [the scrub gowns of the nurses]

3. Irregular plural nouns not ending in *s* need an apostrophe *s* ('s) to form the possessive.

   The *children's* ward is on the fourth floor.

   The *women's* lounge is down the hall.

4. If two people own an item, only the last name takes the possessive form.

   Lorry and Doreen's book on *Grammar and Writing Skills for the Health Professional* is on the shelf.

   If each person owns the item, both names take the possessive form.

   Dr. Archie's and *Dr. Villes's* stethoscopes are on the treatment table.

5. To form the possessive of singular nouns ending in *s*, add an apostrophe and an *s* ('s).

   Mr. Jones's daughter.

6. To form the possessive of plural nouns ending in *s*, add only an apostrophe (').

   The *Jones'* families.

FIGURE 1-5 Rules for Forming Possessive Nouns

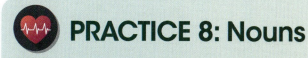

PRACTICE 8: Nouns

Form the possessive of the italicized nouns:

1. The *doctor* examination revealed no fracture. _____

2. The *parent* children showed their concern. _____

3. The *children* dentist is a pedodontist. _____

4. The dental *technician* surgical scrubs are at the office. _____

5. The *pharmacy* location is near the atrium of the hospital. _____

PRACTICE 8: Nouns

Appositives and Direct Address

An *appositive* (APP) is a word or group of words that immediately follows and further identifies another noun. It is usually separated by commas.

 ## Examples

Dr. Villes, *the doctor on call,* performed the endoscopy. [The phrase *the doctor on call* identifies and renames the noun, *Dr. Villes.*]

Oberg Insurance, *an independent firm,* covered all medical expenses. (the phrase *an independent firm* identifies and renames Oberg Insurance.)

The *direct address* (DA) names the listener. The speaker tries to catch the listener's attention by using the person's name. The use of direct address makes messages more direct and personal. Because it interrupts the message, a noun of direct address is separated by commas.

 ## Examples

This equipment, *Miss Archie,* belongs in the treatment room. [The speaker is requesting *Miss Archie* to listen.]

What do you think, *Christopher?* [The speaker is requesting *Christopher* to listen.]

Note that commas separate both appositives and nouns of direct address.

 ## PRACTICE 9: Nouns

Indicate whether the italicized noun or phrase is appositive or direct address by placing APP or DA above it:

1. Tell me, *Doctor,* what is the normal course of treatment for this condition?

2. Do you think, *Dr. Paul,* that the biopsy is necessary?

3. My husband, *Bob,* developed atrial fibrillation.

4. Schedule an appointment, *Pat,* in six months.

5. The assistant, *Laurie,* set the room up for the next patient.

Fill in the blanks below with the correct word from the following group:

direct object	**appositive**	**possessive**	**predicate noun**	**number**
collective noun	**subject noun**	**abstract noun**	**proper noun**	

1. Tells what the sentence is about: _____

2. Names an idea: _____

3. Refers to a group: _____

4. Determines singular or plural: _____

5. Follows a linking verb: _____

6. Receives the verb's action: _____

7. Shows ownership: _____

8. Renames a noun: _____

9. Names a particular person, place, or thing: _____

Identify how the italicized nouns are used in the sentences:

1. *Reports* are dictated by the *physician*. _____

2. The *doctor* gave the *nurse* explicit *directions*. _____

3. *Nurse*, please administer the *medication* now. _____

4. Listen, *Doctor Lee*, the heart is normal. _____

5. *Susan* is the best *nurse* on the *floor*. _____

Nouns Summary

Noun	Names a person, place, thing, or quality.
Common	Names a *class* of persons, places, objects, or qualities: politician, state, author, couple, drug, disease, clinic, company, physician, specimen, virus, therapy, artery, temperature, x-ray.
Proper	Names a *particular* person, place, object, or quality: Republican, Massachusetts, Emily Dickinson, Jack and Jill, Darvon, Hodgkin, Mayo Clinic, Microsoft, Joan Mullins, M.D., Museum of Fine Arts, Basketball Hall of Fame, American Medical Association (AMA), American Association of Medical Assistants (AAMA). Proper nouns are capitalized.
Collective	Names a group of persons, animals, or things: government, association, board, public, society, organization, audience, police, nation, flock.
Abstract	Names a quality or idea not perceived by the senses: honesty, goodness, joy, integrity, honor, worth, value, thought, courage, freedom, fear.
Concrete	Names things that are touchable, visible, and audible: pharmacist, therapist, instrument, forceps, alcohol, ointment, medication, hospital.

Number	Categorizes nouns as singular or plural.
Forming plurals	Add the letter *s* to most nouns: patient, patients; pen, pens; symptom, symptoms; quota, quotas; bone, bones; nurse, nurses.
Nouns ending in *s, x, ch, sh, z*	Add *es*: pass, passes; box, boxes; wish, wishes; index, indexes; quiz, quizzes; phalanx, phalanxes; larynx, larynxes.
Nouns ending in *y* preceded by a *vowel*	Add *s* only: boy, boys; key, keys; attorney, attorneys; delay, delays; donkey, donkeys; Saturday, Saturdays.

Nouns ending in *y* preceded by a *consonant*	Change the *y* to *i* and add *es*: city, cities; allergy, allergies; dictionary, dictionaries; extremity, extremities; dichotomy, dichotomies; deficiency, deficiencies.
Nouns ending in *o* preceded by a *vowel*	Add the letter *s*: studio, studios; shampoo, shampoos; ratio, ratios; stereo, stereos; portfolio, portfolios.
Nouns ending in *o* preceded by a *consonant*	Add *s* or *es*: ego, egos; memo, memos; potato, potatoes; hero, heroes; zero, zeros; auto, autos; typo, typos.
Nouns ending *in f or fe*	Add the letter *s* if the plural form has an *f* sound: belief, beliefs; proof, proofs; safe, safes; staff, staffs. If the plural form has the *v* sound, change the *f* to *v* and add *es*: life, lives; wife, wives; calf, calves; loaf, loaves.
Plurals of Medical Nouns	Make the following changes:
	x to *c* or *g* and add *es*: apex, apices; appendix, appendices; thorax, thoraces; phalanx, phalanges.
	is to *es*: diagnosis, diagnoses; prognosis, prognoses.
	oma to *omata*: stoma, stomata; sarcoma, sarcomata.
	a to *ae*: sequela, sequelae; vertebra, vertebrae.
	um to *a*: ovum, ova; bacterium, bacteria.
	us to *i*: fungus, fungi; streptococcus, streptococci.
	on to *a*: ganglion, ganglia.
	en to *ina*: lumen, lumina.

Function

Categories of usage.

Nominative	Refers to the subject of the sentence about which something is said.
Subject	"The patient receives excellent care." *Receives excellent care* is what is said about the subject, *patient*.
Predicate Noun	Means the same as the subject but comes right after a linking verb. "English is a language." *Language* is the predicate noun that comes after the linking verb, *is*.
Objective	Refers to the object of the sentence or preposition.
Direct Object	Directly receives the action of the verb and answers *who* or *what* about the verb. "Students read [*what*?] books." The direct object is *books*.
Indirect Object	Relates indirectly to the verb and answers *to/for whom* and *to/for what* about the verb. "The physician gave [*to whom*?] the patient [*what*?] a prescription." The *patient* is the indirect object.
Object of a Preposition	Follows a preposition and shows its relationship to the rest of the sentence. "The patient came to the office." *Office* is the object of the preposition *to*.
Possessive	Shows ownership or possession.
Singular	Add an apostrophe and an *s* to singular nouns: ship's name, Chris's truck, month's allotment, boss's approval.
Plural	Add only an apostrophe to plural nouns ending in *s*: boys' games, heroes' medal.
Irregular	Add an apostrophe and an *s*: children's toys, women's blouses.
Appositive	Follows a noun and renames it. "The disease, *an inflammation of the spinal cord and brain*, involves the meninges." Note the separation by commas.
Direct Address	Speaks directly to a person and names the listener. "Listen, *Jane*, to the sounds through the stethoscope." Note the separation by commas.

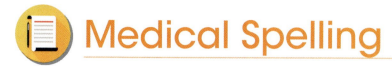

Medical Spelling

Become familiar with the spelling of the following words:

allergy, allergies	diagnosis, diagnoses	ophthalmologist	process, processes
anesthesiologist	embolus, emboli	orthodontist	psychiatrist
anomaly, anomalies	endocrinologist	orthopedist	psychologist
appendix,	extremity,	osteoporosis	psychosomatic
appendices	extremities	otitis	radiologist
bacterium, bacteria	gastroenterologist	otolaryngologist	stratum, strata
biopsy	gynecologist	otologist	symptoms
bronchus, bronchi	immunologist	ovum, ova	thorax, thoraces
cardiologist	medication	pathologist	thrombus, thrombi
deficiency,	neurologist	pharmacist	urologist
deficiencies	nucleus, nuclei	pharmacologist	vertebra, vertebrae
dermatologist	oncologist	physician	

Real-World Applications

Medical Office Correspondence

Correspondence with hand written letters is slowly coming to an end. Computers, emails, smartphones, and linking our encounters and connections are changing. The sophisticated technological computer driven correspondence remains an integral part of the communication system.

In the medical field it is a highly structured form of communication. Correspondence is a process of sharing medical-related information. Through these means, both the receiver and the sender have a document that holds more legality than the spoken word.

The Medical Letter

Medical letters are typed or keyed. They indicate who the letter is from, what is being communicated, and to whom it is being communicated. These typed or keyed sections of a medical letter can provide information about clients, medical records, and other medical concerns at a glance. Since medical letters may pass important and private information from doctor to client, between doctors, or between facilities and insurance companies, it is important that the appearance of the medical letter reflect competence by utilizing correct formatting and organization to facilitate communication.

Medical assistants very often have to assist and communicate with written letters. The appearance and quality of the letter is a reflection of the medical assistant and his or her employer. Sentences should be concise and short. Any correspondence should also be accurate and courteous. Spelling should be checked, rechecked, and proofread. Many English medical spell check programs correct misspelled words but may not be accurate. The style and format of the correspondence is determined by the employer.

There are four basic letter styles used by medical personnel.

1. Full Block

2. Modified Block (standard)

3. Semi-Modified Block (indented)
4. Simplified

Full Block

- In a *full block letter*, all lines are flush with the left margin. This is the quickest, most efficient, and least confusing style of letter.
- The date is usually printed on line 15, or *two to three lines* below the heading.
- The inside address is flush to the left margin, *four lines* below the date and may be three or four lines in length.
- The salutation is flush to the left margin and on the *second line* below the inside address.
- If there is a subject line it is on the *second line* below the salutation, flush to the left margin. The subject line is optional. It indicates the purpose of the letter. It is often prefaced with "Subject:" or "Re:" to distinguish it from the body of the letter.
- The body of the letter begins *two lines* below the salutation.
- The complimentary closing is on the *second line* below the body of the letter.
- The typed or keyed signature is *four lines* below the complimentary closing, leaving space for the written or signed letter.
- Reference initials are below the typed or keyed signature with the individual's initials who composed the letter in UPPER CASE and the medical assistant's initials who typed or keyed the letter in lower case.

    Figure 1-6 presents an example of a block style letter.

Modified Block (Standard)

In a *modified block (standard) letter*, all of the lines are flush to the left margin except for the date and complimentary closing with signature.

Figure 1-7 presents an example of a modified block style letter.

Semi-Modified Block (Indented)

In a *semi-modified block (indented) letter*, the first line of every paragraph is indented five spaces.

Figure 1-8 presents an example of a semi-modified block style letter.

Simplified

In a *simplified letter*, there is no salutation or complimentary closure. All of the lines are flush to the left margin. This style is most often used with form letters written from a template. They are usually intended for a wide audience.

Figure 1-9 presents an example of a simplified style letter.

Letter Components

Heading

The letterhead is usually commercially printed with a logo. When using letterhead paper, only the date needs to be typed. The date is placed *two to three lines* below the letterhead, flush with the left margin (Figure 1-10).

V
M   VILLES MEDICAL CENTER
C   *One Morey Place*
Anywhere, MA 01102
(555) 555-4727 Phone
(555) 555-4000 Fax

July 15, 20XX

Dr. Valerie Christopher
Carr and Oberg Associates
25 Brewster Street
Anywhere, MA 01518

Dear Dr. Christopher:

Thank you for referring your patient, Mr. Burt Weaver, to Villes Medical Center. Mr. Weaver's psychological status on his initial evaluation necessitated an emergency evaluation. I diagnosed the patient as having an adjustment disorder and major depression. He was placed on antidepressant medication for three months.

During this time, Mr. Weaver also participated in six group sessions and ten individual psychotherapy sessions before reaching his maximum rehabilitation. At the time of his discharge, Mr. Weaver was made aware that he could return to Villes Medical Center at any time, if warranted.

If you have any further questions, please call my office at (555) 555-4727.

Yours truly,

Dr. Mary Louis Norman

LNV

FIGURE 1-6 Block Style Letter

V
M
C

VILLES MEDICAL CENTER
One Morey Place
Anywhere, MA 01102
(555) 555-4727 Phone
(555) 555-4000 Fax

July 15, 20XX

Dr. Valerie Christopher
Carr and Oberg Associates
25 Brewster Street
Anywhere, MA 01518

Dear Dr. Christopher:

Thank you for referring your patient, Mr. Burt Weaver, to Villes Medical Center. Mr. Weaver's psychological status on his initial evaluation necessitated an emergency evaluation. I diagnosed the patient as having an adjustment disorder and major depression. He was placed on antidepressant medication for three months.

During this time, Mr. Weaver also participated in six group sessions and ten individual psychotherapy sessions before reaching his maximum rehabilitation. At the time of his discharge, Mr. Weaver was made aware that he could return to Villes Medical Center at any time, if warranted.

If you have any further questions, please call my office at (555) 555-4727.

Yours truly,

Dr. Mary Louis Norman

LNV

FIGURE 1-7 Modified Block Letter

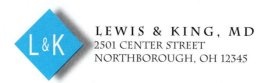

LEWIS & KING, MD
2501 CENTER STREET
NORTHBOROUGH, OH 12345

NORTHBOROUGH
FAMILY MEDICAL GROUP

January 12, 20XX (approximately 15th line)

Jeremy Brown, MD   (approximately 20th line)
111 S Main
Blossom, UT 10283-1120

Dear Dr. Brown:

Blossom Medical Society Meeting

Thank you for inviting me to speak at the Blossom Medical Society Meeting June 15, 20XX. As requested, my topic will describe the use of the MRI in assisting physicians to make a more accurate diagnosis without resorting to invasive procedures. The exact title of my speech will be sent by next Friday.

Please have your office manager send information regarding the number of participants expected, time of meeting, location, and any other details that will assist me in preparing my speech.

I will write or call if I have any additional questions.

Yours truly,

Winston Lewis, MD

Winston Lewis, MD

WL:jg

Enclosure: Handout on MRI

FIGURE 1-8 Semi-Modified Block Letter

Inside Address

The inside address gives the name and address of the person or facility to which the letter is going. It is the mailing address. It is flush with the left margin (Figure 1-11).

If the title of the person is included in the inside address, it goes after the name on the same line.

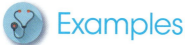

Examples

Dr. Valerie Christopher, President
Carr and Oberg Associates
25 Brewster Street
Anywhere, MA 00000-1111

Mary Louise Norman, M.D.
Chairperson, Board of Directors
25 Brewster Street
Anywhere, MA 00000-1111

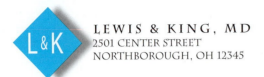

LEWIS & KING, MD
2501 CENTER STREET
NORTHBOROUGH, OH 12345

NORTHBOROUGH
FAMILY MEDICAL GROUP

January 12, 20XX (app.roximately 15th line)

Jeremy Brown, MD   (approximately 20th line)
111 S Main
Blossom, UT 10283-1120

(triple-space)

Blossom Medical Society Meeting

(triple-space)

Thank you for inviting me to speak at the Blossom Medical Society Meeting June 15, 20XX. As requested, my topic will describe the use of the MRI in assisting physicians to make a more accurate diagnosis without resorting to invasive procedures. The exact title of my speech will be sent by next Friday.

Please have your office manager send information regarding the number of participants expected, time of meeting, location, and any other details that will assist me in preparing my speech.

I will write or call if I have any additional questions.

Winston Lewis, MD   (4 line spaces)

Winston Lewis, MD

WL:jg

Enclosure: Handout on MRI

FIGURE 1-9 Simplified Letter

V
M
C
VILLES MEDICAL CENTER
One Morey Place
Anywhere, MA 01102
(555) 555-4727 Phone
(555) 555-4000 Fax

July 15, 20XX

FIGURE 1-10 Heading

VMC

VILLES MEDICAL CENTER
One Morey Place
Anywhere, MA 01102
(555) 555-4727 Phone
(555) 555-4000 Fax

July 15, 20XX

Dr. Valerie Christopher
Carr and Oberg Associates
25 Brewster Street
Anywhere, MA 01518

FIGURE 1-11 Inside Address

Salutation

The salutation is the greeting of the letter. It is placed *two lines* below the inside address, flush with the left margin. A colon (:) follows the salutation (Figure 1-12). All words in the salutation begin with capital letters, except articles and prepositions.

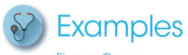 Examples

Firm or Group	Dear Customer Service Representative, Colleagues, Friends, Members of the Search Committee, Gentlemen, Ladies, Editors, Physicians, Students
Special Unknown Person	Dear Personnel Director, Sir, Madame, Clerk of Deeds, Nurse Supervisor
Special Known Persons	Dear Dr. Norman, Nurse Rose, Mr. Oberg, Mary, Miss Leclaire

VMC

VILLES MEDICAL CENTER
One Morey Place
Anywhere, MA 01102
(555) 555-4727 Phone
(555) 555-4000 Fax

July 15, 20XX

Dr. Valerie Christopher
Carr and Oberg Associates
25 Brewster Street
Anywhere, MA 01518

Dear Dr. Christopher:

FIGURE 1-12 Salutation

Subject line

If a subject line is used, it is used to call attention to what is important in the letter (Figure 1-13). The subject line is optional. It indicates the purpose of the letter. It is often prefaced with "Subject:" or "Re:" to distinguish it from the body of the letter. The subject line is keyed or typed *two lines* below the salutation. It is flush to the left margin.

V
M VILLES MEDICAL CENTER
C *One Morey Place*
Anywhere, MA 01102
(555) 555-4727 Phone
(555) 555-4000 Fax

July 15, 20XX

Dr. Valerie Christopher
Carr and Oberg Associates
25 Brewster Street
Anywhere, MA 01518

Mr. Burt Weaver

Dear Dr. Christopher:

Thank you for referring. . . .

FIGURE 1-13 Use of Subject Line

Body

The body of the letter contains the message. The body may have more than one paragraph with double spacing between each paragraph (Figure 1-14).

Complimentary Closing and Signature

The closing is the leave-taking part of the letter (Figure 1-15). It is typed on the *second line* below the last line of the body. Only the first word in the closing is capitalized. A comma is placed after the last word.

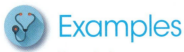

Examples

Yours truly,	Sincerely,	Thank you,
Very truly yours,	Sincerely yours,	With best wishes,
With best regards,	Cordially,	Respectfully yours,

VILLES MEDICAL CENTER
One Morey Place
Anywhere, MA 01102
(555) 555-4727 Phone
(555) 555-4000 Fax

July 15, 20XX

Dr. Valerie Christopher
Carr and Oberg Associates
25 Brewster Street
Anywhere, MA 01518

Dear Dr. Christopher:

Thank you for referring your patient, Mr. Burt Weaver, to Villes Medical Center. Mr. Weaver's psychological status on his initial evaluation necessitated an emergency evaluation. I diagnosed the patient as having an adjustment disorder and major depression. He was placed on antidepressant medication for three months.

During this time, Mr. Weaver also participated in six group sessions and ten individual psychotherapy sessions before reaching his maximum rehabilitation. At the time of his discharge, Mr. Weaver was made aware that he could return to Villes Medical Center at any time, if warranted.

If you have any further questions, please call my office at (555) 555-4727.

FIGURE 1-14 Body

The signature is *directly below* the closing.

Keyed or Typed Signature

The writer's name is keyed or typed *four lines* directly below the closing. In some letters it may be *six lines* below the complimentary closing. The keyed or typed name may also include the writer's position.

Reference Initials, Enclosures, and Copy Notations

The author's initials are keyed or typed in capital letters with the medical assistant's initials following in lower case. It is flush with the left margin. Enclosures are *one or two lines* below the reference initials. It is keyed or typed with an "Enc." If copies of a letter are given to other people, "C:" and the name of the person to whom the copy is sent should be typed on a new line following "Enc," or the typist's initials.

V
M
C

VILLES MEDICAL CENTER
One Morey Place
Anywhere, MA 01102
(555) 555-4727 Phone
(555) 555-4000 Fax

July 15, 20XX

Dr. Valerie Christopher
Carr and Oberg Associates
25 Brewster Street
Anywhere, MA 01518

Dear Dr. Christopher:

Thank you for referring your patient, Mr. Burt Weaver, to Villes Medical Center. Mr. Weaver's psychological status on his initial evaluation necessitated an emergency evaluation. I diagnosed the patient as having an adjustment disorder and major depression. He was placed on antidepressant medication for three months.

During this time, Mr. Weaver also participated in six group sessions and ten individual psychotherapy sessions before reaching his maximum rehabilitation. At the time of his discharge, Mr. Weaver was made aware that he could return to Villes Medical Center at any time, if warranted.

If you have any further questions, please call my office at (555) 555-4727.

Yours truly,

Dr. Mary Louis Norman

FIGURE 1-15 Closing and Signature

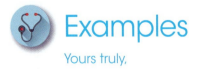 **Examples**

Yours truly,

Dr. Mary Louis Norman

LNV

Enc.

C: Mary Pat Leonard, M.D.

If the office's name and address do not appear at the top of the stationery, key or type this information under the writer's typed name (or title) following the signature.

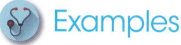 Examples

Dr. Mary Louis Norman   Anywhere, MA 00000-1111

Villes Medical Center   (555) 555-5555

One Morey Place   (555) 555-0000 Fax

Heading on the Second Page

If a letter runs longer than one page, the heading on the second page should contain the name of the writer, the page number, and the date. It should begin flush with the left margin.

 Examples

(1)   Mary Louis Norman, M.D.   -2-   July 15, 20XX

(2)   Mary Louis Norman, M.D.   Page 2   July 15, 20XX

(3)   Mary Louis Norman, M.D.   Page 2   July 15, 20XX

Subject: Mr. Burt Weaver

 PRACTICE 10: Parts of a Letter

Match the terms with their definitions:

1. body _____   A. leave-taking of the letter

2. written signature _____   B. typed name of sender

3. heading _____   C. the greeting

4. closing _____   D. parts of the letter are indented

5. inside address _____   E. everything in letter begins at the left margin

6. letterhead stationery _____   F. company's name and address printed on stationery

7. typed signature _____   G. message of the letter

8. block style letter _____   H. person and address to whom the letter is written

9. salutation _____   I. address of the person writing the letter

Addressing Envelopes

Envelopes can be inserted in the printers selecting the envelope format on the software. Labels may be used and adhered to the envelope. The address should be typed or printed in all capital letters. A return address should be in the upper left-hand corner of the envelope, typed, printed, or preprinted. Information for the post office, such as "Certified," is usually printed under the stamp. Information for the addressee, such as "Personal" or "Private," is written under the return address (Figure 1-16).

The automated machines read addresses of mail from the bottom up and will look for the city, state, and ZIP code first. If the automated machine cannot read it properly, the mail will be destroyed or misrouted.

The U.S. Postal Service (USPS) suggests these points and tips:

- All capital letters
- No punctuation
- At least 10-point type
- One space between the city and state
- Two spaces between the state and ZIP code
- Simple type fonts
- The address is justified to the left
- Black ink on white or light paper
- If the address is inside a window, make sure there is at least 1/8 inch clearance around the address (so that parts of the address don't slip out of view, making the address unreadable to the mail processing machines).
- If using labels, make sure you do not cut off any important information. Make sure they are on straight as the automated machines have trouble reading slanted info.

Other tips from the U.S. Postal Service:

- Always put the attention line on top of—never below—the city and state on the bottom.
- If you can't put the suite or apartment number on the same line as the delivery address, put it on the line above, not the line below.
- East and west are very important directions in an address.

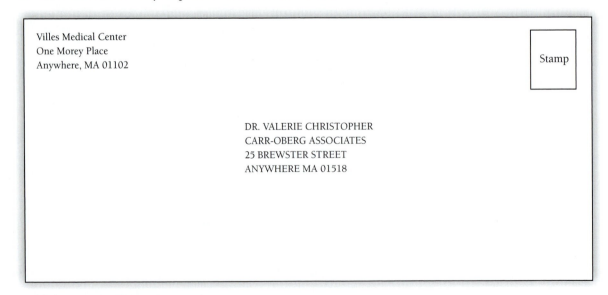

FIGURE 1-16 Addressing the Envelope

- Twenty-five percent of mail pieces have something wrong … for instance, a missing number or wrong ZIP code. They may be delivered, but it costs the postal service time and money.

- If the first class mail is square or rigid or meets one of the non-machinable characteristics, it will be subject to surcharge.

- Fancy fonts are often not readable.

- No patterns or glossy envelopes. The paper should be white or light in color to be read by the automated machine.

- Further information can be found at usps.com

Folding the Letter

Place the letter face down, folding the letter into equal thirds or in an S shape pattern (Figure 1-17). Before creasing the two lines, be sure the edges meet. Some people use a ruler to make neater creases.

Be sure the envelope is addressed before putting the folded letter into the envelope. Also, be sure the top of the letter is at the top of the envelope.

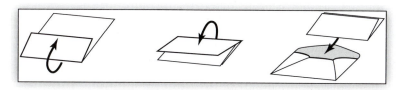

FIGURE 1-17   Folding the Business Letter

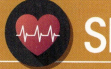 ## Skills Review

Write the noun usage for the italicized word(s) in each sentence: **S** *for subject,* **DO** *for direct object,* **IO** *for indirect object,* **OP** *for object of preposition,* **APP** *for appositive,* **PN** *for predicate noun, and* **DA** *for direct address.*

1. The left *knee* was limited in motion due to intrinsic pathology.

2. Hillside Medical Associates pays its *employees* competitive *salaries*.

3. Most *physicians* read several *journals* each week.

4. The *AMA* will hold its *election* next month.

5. *Visualization* of the *joint* is done with an *endoscope*.

6. The medical *assistant* transcribed the *report* for the *doctor*.

7. *Nurse*, would you please check my *temperature*?

8. *Muscles* can perform a variety of *actions*.

9. *Cramps* are painful *contractions* of *muscles*.

10. The *calcaneus* is the heel *bone*.

Rewrite these sentences correcting capitals, spellings, possessives, and plurals where necessary.

1. Dr. smith is on call for orthopedic consultation.

   _____

2. Bones cannot move without the help of muscles'.

   _____

3. the admitting diagnosis is acute intertrochanteric fracture of the Right Hip.

   _____

4. Copys of the report were mailed to the patients physician.

   _____

5. Thousands of patients spread bacterium to other workers.

   _____

If the noun in italic print is singular, make it plural. If the noun is plural, make it singular.

1. The patient had multiple *diagnosis*. _____

2. The bacterium responsible for the disease is the *gonococci*. _____

3. The outer layer of skin has cells that are arranged in *stratum*. _____

4. In a colostomy, the proximal *stomata* drains the feces. _____

5. Many *villus* in the small intestines absorb nutrients. _____

6. Diverticulosis is saclike swellings present in the wall of the colon called *diverticulum*. _____

7. The blocking of a coronary artery by *thrombi* could lead to an M.I. _____

Change proper nouns in italics to common nouns and common nouns in italics to proper nouns.

1. The *patient* expects and appreciates courtesy. _____

2. Due to an accident, *James* has a greenstick fracture of the right ulna.
   _____

3. The *doctor* praised the *medical assistant* for her efficiency. _____

4. The *AMA* is a prestigious group. _____

5. Most doctors send their patients to the *Mayo Clinic*. _____

6. The *hospital* hired a new *specialist*. _____

Identify the medical nouns in the following sentences:

1. Health information coding is transferring the description of disease, injuries, and procedures into letters and numbers (alphanumeric).

2. Congenital anomaly is a birth defect.

3. The symptoms are similar to a myocardial infarction.

4. Otitis media is common in young patients.

5. The dermatologist wants a biopsy sent to the pathologist.

Indicate whether these statements are true or false.

1. The modified block style letter has no indentation.

2. "Yours truly" is a common salutation in a medical letter.

3. "C" in a letter means a copy was sent to an additional person/s.

4. The number of folds for an 8½-inch by 11-inch paper is three.

5. "Re:" and "Subject:" have the same meaning.

Circle the correct plural form of these words. If necessary, check a medical dictionary.

1. antenna   antennas, antenni, antennae

2. extremity   extremities, extremites, extremmities

3. metamorphosis   metamorphos, metamorphos, metamorphoses

4. bacterium   bacteria, bacteri, bacteriac

5. symptom   symptam, symptim, symptoms

6. anomaly   anomilies, anomalys, anomalies

7. diaphysis   diaphysises, diaphyses, diaphysiss

8. vertebra   vertebrum, vertebrae, vertebri

9. process   processes, processos, processs

10. Phalanx   phalanxes, phalanges, phalanxs

11. diagnosis   diagnoss, diagnosiss, diagnosing, diagnoses

12. ganglion   ganglionss, ganglia, gangli

 # Comprehensive Review

Match these words with the corresponding numbers found in the letter (Figure 1-18).

a. appositive
b. salutation
c. direct object

d. object of a preposition
e. proper noun

f. subject
g. closing
h. predicate noun

i. inside address
j. common noun

1. _____   4. _____   7. _____   10. _____

2. _____   5. _____   8. _____

3. _____   6. _____   9. _____

LINCOLN MEDICAL OFFICE
1 VASSER STREET
BOSTON, MA 05440

June 14, 20XX

Dr. William Ward
5609 Main Street   ⎫
②   ⎬ ①
Boston, MA 05402-0000 ⎭

Dear Dr. Ward: ③

Thank you for referring your *patient*, *Ms. Emily Parker*, to this office. My diagnosis of this woman was
major *depression*. I prescribed *an antidepressant* for a period of three months. *Ms. Parker* will return in
September for a follow-up *appointment*. Call me if you have any questions.

Sincerely,   ⑩

Dr. Peter Morin

Dr. Peter Morin

FIGURE 1-18   Letter for comprehensive review

SECTION 2
Pronouns
Practical Writing Component: Emails and Memos

Objectives

After reading this section, the learner should be able to:

- identify basic types of pronouns
- identify personal pronouns by gender, number, and function
- use pronouns that agree with their antecedents in number, gender, and person
- spell various medical terms
- compose an office memorandum and email

 # Introduction

Once upon a time there was a medical office unit with four medical assistants named *Everybody, Somebody, Anybody,* and *Nobody.* There was an important job to be done, and *Everybody* was sure that *Somebody* would do it. *Anybody* could have done it, but *Nobody* did it. *Somebody* got angry with this because it was *Everybody's* job. *Everybody* thought *Anybody* could do it, but *Nobody* realized that *Everybody* wouldn't do it. It ended up that *Everybody* blamed *Somebody* when *Nobody* did what *Anybody* could have done. (Author unknown)

Welcome to the world of pronouns. A *pronoun* is a word that replaces or substitutes for a noun; for example,

Leah borrowed *books* from the library. *She* returned *them* yesterday.

Note that the pronouns *she* and *them take* the place of the nouns *Leah* and *books.* Because of the close relationship between nouns and pronouns, there are a lot of similarities in how both are used in sentences. Therefore, anyone with a good understanding of nouns will have no difficulty with pronouns.

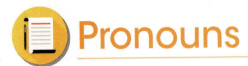
Pronouns

The different types of pronouns are personal, reflexive, relative, indefinite, interrogative, and demonstrative. The meaning of each pronoun is contained within its name, which makes the definitions easier to understand:

- Personal pronouns refer to persons (and things).
- Reflexive pronouns throw back or reflect.
- Relative pronouns relate to other words.
- Indefinite pronouns refer to the unknown.
- Interrogative pronouns ask questions.
- Demonstrative pronouns point out or demonstrate.

Personal Pronouns

Personal pronouns refer to specific people and things. They are used more frequently than any other pronoun. Personal pronouns have three characteristics: gender, number, and person. They are also distinguished by case, being either nominative, objective, or possessive. Choosing which personal pronoun to use depends on how it is used in a sentence.

Personal Pronouns

I, you, he, she, it, we, you, they,
me, you, him, her, it, us, you, them, my, mine, your,
yours, his, her, hers, its, our, ours, your, yours, their, theirs

---

Gender

Pronouns are characterized by gender: masculine, feminine, neuter, and indefinite. Masculine pronouns are *he, his, him.* Feminine pronouns are *she, her, hers.* The word *it* is an example of a neuter pronoun. Indefinite pronouns represent unknown persons or things, such as *all, anything, someone.*

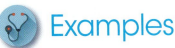
Examples

He is very protective of *his* property. [masculine]

Anyone can be successful. [indefinite]

It belongs to the person who finds *it,* I believe. [neuter]

She was all ears after *she* learned about *her* grades. [feminine]

Number and Person

Number shows whether a pronoun refers to one person or thing (singular) or more than one (plural). Person denotes whether one is speaking (first person), spoken to (second person), or spoken about (third person). Table 2-1 shows pronoun forms categorized by person and number.

		Number	
Person	**Meaning**	**Singular**	**Plural**
First	Speaker	I, me, my, mine	we, us, our, ours
Second	Individual addressed	you, your, yours	you, your, yours
Third	Person or thing spoken about	he, she, it, its, him, his, her, hers	they, them, their, theirs

TABLE 2-1   Number and Person of Pronouns

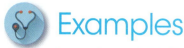 Examples

I am always right. [first person singular]

We are at the medical conference. [first person plural]

My schedule is very busy. [first person singular]

You should check the treatment room for antiseptics. [second person singular or plural]

You make *your* own way. [second person singular or plural]

He said the matter could be settled now. [third person singular]

They should have signed the medical consent form. [third person plural]

The anatomy books belong to *them*. [third person plural]

 PRACTICE 1: Number and Person

Use Table 2-1 to identify the italicized pronouns in the following sentences as first, second, or third person and singular or plural:

1. The exam took a long time but *it* was simple. _____

2. As nurses, *we* need to help lessen health care disparities. _____

3. Are they *your* new patients? _____

4. The medical history given to *us* was complete. _____

5. *They* found a kidney stone in the strainer. _____

Nominative Case (Subject)

The choice of pronouns depends on how they function in a sentence, which heads to the explanation of case. The subject pronoun—*I, you, he, she, it, we,* and *they*—is the person or thing talked about in a sentence.

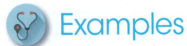 Examples

He tripped on the stairs.

They work at the Medical Center.

She is the Chief Resident.

I felt confident I could do the job.

Although the bronchoscopy was simple, *it* took a long time to do.

 PRACTICE 2: Nominative Case – Subject

Choose the correct pronoun from within the parentheses:

1. Dr. Jones, (you, your) have no idea how much work is involved in preparing the patient.
2. (She, Her) answered the office telephone immediately.
3. (It, Its) doesn't make any difference what the EKG reads.
4. As a medical group, (we, us) support our diagnosis.
5. Studies indicate (it, its) takes 4–6 doses before the symptoms disappear.

Nominative Case (Predicate)

Predicate pronouns are the same as subject pronouns: *I, you, he, she, it, we,* and *they.* They are found following a linking verb such as am, is, are, was, or were.

 Examples

The visitor must have been *she.*

Is *she* the owner?

Is it *I*?

It is *she* who pays the bill.

Was it *he* who called?

 PRACTICE 3: Nominative Case – Predicate

Choose the correct predicate pronoun from within the parentheses:

1. It was (me, I) who administered cardiopulmonary resuscitation.
2. The resident who did the physical exam on the patients was (he, him).
3. Is it (she, her) who has the diagnosis of hypertension?
4. The cholecystectomy patient is (it, she).
5. Born in a foreign country, (them, they) felt fearful and uneasy in the hospital.

Objective Case

A pronoun naming the person or thing that receives the action of the verb either directly or indirectly is an object pronoun.

The direct object pronoun—*me, you, him, her, it, us, you,* and *them*—receives the action of the sentence.

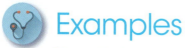
Examples

The patient paid *them* in cash.

Laurie helped *me* with the amniocentesis.

The indirect object pronoun, like the noun, receives the indirect action of the verb. It names the person **to** or **for whom** something is done, or **to** or **for what** something is done.

The indirect object pronouns are the same as the object pronouns: *me, you, him, her, it, us, you,* and *them.*

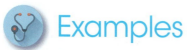
Examples

Dr. Rodriguez gave *you* some medication.

The change in surgical procedures saved *them* time.

The AMA loaned *us* medical literature.

Evelyn sent *me* the x-ray report.

Pronouns that follow a preposition are also objective: *me, you, him, her, it, us, you,* and *them.*

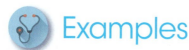
Examples

I gave the sphygmomanometer to *them.*

Jane spoke to *her* several times on the phone.

It was a good thing for *them* to do.

English is taught to *her* and *me.*

Possessive Case

The *possessive case* shows ownership or possession. The possessive pronouns are *my, mine, your, yours, his, her, hers, our, ours, their,* and *theirs.* Table 2-2 summarizes the various cases of pronouns.

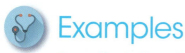
Examples

The patient refused to eat *his* food.

The blue lab coat is *mine.*

The urinalysis is *hers.*

TABLE 2-2	Cases of Personal Pronouns	
Nominative Case	**Objective Case**	**Possessive Case**
Subject and predicate pronouns: I, you, he, she, it, we, they	Direct and indirect object or object of a preposition: me, you, him, her, it, us, you, them	Possessive pronouns: my, mine, your, yours, his, her, hers, its, our, ours, their, theirs

 # PRACTICE 4: Cases of Pronouns

Select the correct pronoun from within the parentheses. State how it is used in each sentence: subject, predicate, direct object, indirect object, object of a preposition, or possessive.

1. (He, Me) had no idea about the aneurysm. _____
2. I carried a stethoscope with (me, I). _____
3. (Them, They) should get the electrocardiogram from (he, him). _____
4. (Her, Hers) bronchoscopy showed carcinoma of the lungs. _____
5. Is (she, her) doing the urinalysis? _____

Reflexive Pronouns

Reflexive pronouns reflect back to the person. The pronoun refers to a noun or pronoun that appears earlier in the sentence. To form them, add *self or selves* to the personal pronoun. Depending on how it is used in the sentence, a reflexive pronoun can be a direct object, indirect object, object of a preposition, or a predicate pronoun.

> **Reflexive Pronouns**
>
> myself, yourself, himself, herself, itself, ourselves, themselves

 ## Examples

She buys *herself* a stethoscope. [indirect object]

He gives *himself* insulin injections every day. [indirect object]

I am *myself* only when I feel good. [predicate pronoun after the linking verb *am*]

They smiled at *themselves* when the procedure was over. [object of a preposition]

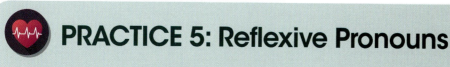

PRACTICE 5: Reflexive Pronouns

Provide the correct reflexive pronoun:

1. Doreen and Val enjoyed _____.
2. Laurie volunteered the information _____.
3. Ms. Ville did the procedure _____.
4. Dr. Archie gave _____ an hour to complete the amniocentesis.
5. Charlie canceled the appointments _____.

Relative Pronouns

Relative pronouns relate one part of a sentence to a word in another part of the sentence.

A relative pronoun helps to join a relative clause to the rest of the sentence. The most important relative pronouns are *who, which,* and *that.*

Who refers to people.

Relative Pronouns
who, whom, whose, which, what, that

 ## Examples

The patient *who* needs the antiemetic is in room 430.

Who is the relative pronoun that refers to the patient.

The physician *who* ordered the procedure is on rounds.

Which refers to things. *Which* is used when the clause that it introduces is not essential to the meaning of the sentence.

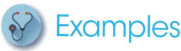 ## Examples

The medical record, *which* is confidential, shows the diagnosis.

The crash cart, *which* is used for emergencies, needs to be restocked.

That refers to people or things. *That* is used when the clause that it introduces is essential to the meaning of the sentence.

PRACTICE 6: Relative Pronouns

 ## Examples

The type *that* is needed for this wound is a figure eight bandage.

The doctor wrote the letter *that* has the information.

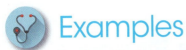 ## PRACTICE 6: Relative Pronouns

Select the correct pronoun:

1. The patient has Dr. Villes, (who, that) is scheduled to go on vacation tomorrow.
2. Diagnostic tests, (which, who) are used for cardiopathy, should be read by a cardiologist.
3. This is the telemetry (which, that) records the heart rate.
4. Progress notes (who, that) are documented in various styles are legal documents.
5. The patient had cryotherapy (who, that) included cold compresses.

Indefinite Pronouns

Indefinite pronouns refer to persons or things in general. Most indefinite pronouns are singular and require a singular verb.

Indefinite Pronouns

all, another, any, anybody, anyone, anything, both, each, each one, either, everybody, everyone, everything, few, many, most, much, neither, nobody, none, no one, nothing, one, other, several, some, somebody, someone, something, such

---

 ## Examples

Each of the employees wants [singular verb] *her* surgical scrubs ordered through the catalog.

Anyone who gives [singular verb] to charity is twice blessed.

Neither person knows [singular verb] the correct answer.

Every pharmaceutical company has *its* own sales person.

Everyone will send *his/her* consultation to the medical team by Friday.

Some indefinite pronouns are always plural, such as *many, several, few, these,* and *those.* The indefinite pronouns *this, that, each, either,* and *neither* are always singular.

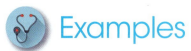 Examples

Many on the medical staff expressed *their* concerns about the care given to patients.

Several voiced *their* anger.

All staff members are to report to *their* stations.

Neither nurse wants to change shifts.

The indefinite pronouns *all, some, any,* and *none* are either singular or plural depending on the number of the noun to which they refer.

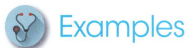 Examples

None of the equipment is [singular verb] modern.

All the students knew *their* [plural verb] abbreviations by heart.

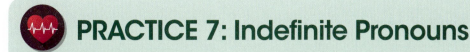 PRACTICE 7: Indefinite Pronouns

Write S if the pronoun is singular and P if the pronoun is plural:

1. Either of the girls can perform her procedure. _____

2. Each of the PDRs was returned to its proper place. _____

3. Many of the assistants brought their dictation equipment. _____

4. Both raised their quality standards. _____

5. Few of the pharmacies wanted their prices to increase. _____

PRACTICE 7: Indefinite Pronouns

Interrogative Pronouns

Interrogative pronouns are used simply to ask questions. They are *who, whom, whose, which,* and *what.* Note that these pronouns are also relative.

Interrogative Pronouns

who, whom, whose, which, what

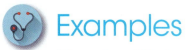 Examples

Who ordered this type of medication?

What caused the fever?

Demonstrative Pronouns

The easiest pronouns to learn are the *demonstrative pronouns*: *this*, *that*, *these*, and *those*. They point out. The pronouns *this* (singular) and *these* (plural) point out people or things that are near in space or time. The pronouns *that* (singular) and *those* (plural) refer to people or things that are farther away in space or time.

Demonstrative Pronouns

this, that, these, those

When writing, place a noun close to the demonstrative pronoun to make the sentence clearer.

 ## Examples

This is the first restaurant on the street. [The demonstrative pronoun *this* points out the *restaurant*.]

These need sterilizing.

That was a good decision.

Those are rare tumors.

 ## PRACTICE 8: Interrogative and Demonstrative Pronouns

Identify the pronouns as demonstrative or interrogative:

1. This needs to be filed in the medical records. _____

2. These are the suture scissors. _____

3. Which is your health insurance plan? _____

4. Those are found with the retractors. _____

5. Who read the EKG? _____

PRACTICE 9: Personal Pronouns

Identify each pronoun as personal, reflexive, relative, indefinite, interrogative, or demonstrative:

1. The medical report was given to me to transcribe. _____

2. Who would think the illness was a malignancy? _____

3. We have to sterilize the instruments ourselves. _____

4. The doctor examined his patient. _____

5. I didn't know the etiology of the disease. _____

Pronoun-Antecedent Agreement

The noun that a pronoun replaces is called its *antecedent*. All pronouns have noun antecedents. The antecedent usually appears before the pronoun.

Bill applied an *antiseptic. He* applied *it.* [*Bill* is the antecedent for the pronoun *he,* and *antiseptic* is the antecedent for the pronoun *it.*]

Pronouns may also be antecedents of other pronouns.

He took *his* antibiotics. [*He* is the antecedent of *his.*]

Pronouns must agree with their noun antecedents in three ways: number, gender, and person.

Number

Use a singular pronoun to refer to a singular noun.

Alice wants *her* report finished today. [*Alice* and *her* are singular.]

Use plural pronouns to refer to plural nouns.

The *Smiths* are giving a party at *their* home. [*Smiths* and *their* are plural.]

When antecedents are joined by *or* or *nor,* the pronoun agrees with the antecedent nearest to the pronoun.

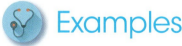

Examples

Neither Jim nor the *assistants* want *their* positions taken away. [The word *assistants* is closer and plural, so the plural pronoun *their* is used.]

Either Mary or *Ellen* wants to do *her* share.

Use a plural pronoun when two antecedents are joined by the word *and.*

Harry and I think *we* need a raise in pay.

Gender

Use masculine, feminine, or neuter pronouns depending on the gender of their antecedents.

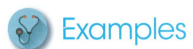

Examples

The man *brought* his *antibiotics to work.* [Man *and* his *are masculine.*]

Mary increased her *skills with practice.* [Mary *and* her *are feminine.*]

The tracing *is irregular;* it *shows artifacts.* [Tracing *and* it *are neuter.*]

When in doubt about the gender, two options are possible:

1. Use *his/her:* One of the students bought *his or her* book.
2. Make the noun plural and use the plural pronoun: *Students* bought *their* books.

Commonly Confused Pronouns: The Use of Its and It's

It   Used only to refer to a specific noun: "When the *code alarm* rings, *it* can be heard a mile away."

Its   The possessive pronoun: "The *stethoscope* is missing *its* diaphragm."

It's   The contraction for "it is." The apostrophe is the sign that the word is used as a contraction: "*it's* a normal EKG" means "*it is* a normal EKG."

One way to check the correct usage of "it's" is to say *it is* instead when reading the sentence. For example, in "The computer printed (it's, its) hardcopy," using *it's* would make it read: "The computer printed *it is* hardcopy." That is not correct. The possessive, *its*, shows that the computer owns the hardcopy, and that is the correct form of the pronoun to use.

PRACTICE 10: Antecedents

Identify the antecedent of the pronoun in each sentence:

1. The doctor wrote *his* cerebrovascular article. _____

2. The patient corrected *his* insulin injection. _____

3. Val and I practiced *our* medical terminology. _____

4. Pat wondered if *she* qualified. _____

5. Medical personnel should know *their* CPR technique. _____

Select the correct pronoun from within the parentheses:

1. Bill and (she, her) went to (her, their) class on cardiopulmonary resuscitation.

2. When a patient has a cerebrovascular accident, (they, she/he) may become hemiplegic.

3. Some people develop hypertension as (they, his/her) get older.

4. They plan to explain (their, them) reasons for diagnosing pancreatitis.

5. Can you and the committee give us (their, them) decision?

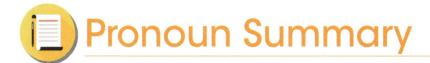

Pronoun Summary

Pronoun	**A word that replaces or substitutes for a noun.**
Personal	Refers to persons. *Singular:* I, me, my, mine, you, your, yours, he, she, it, him, her, his, hers, its. *Plural:* we, us, our, ours, you, your, yours, they, them, their, theirs.
Reflexive	Reflects, throws back: myself, yourself, himself, herself, itself, ourselves, themselves.
Relative	Relates to other words: who, whom, whose, which, what, that, whomever, whichever, whatever.
Indefinite	Refers to persons or things in general: all, another, any, anybody, anyone, anything, both, each, each one, either, everybody, everyone, everything, few, many, most, much, neither, nobody, none, no one, nothing, one, other, several, some, somebody, someone, something, such.
Interrogative	Asks questions: who, whom, whose, which, what.
Demonstrative	Points out, demonstrates: this, that, these, those.

Usage Forms

	Subjective (subject)	Objective (object)	Possessive with Noun	Possessive without Noun	Reflexive (same person or thing as subject)
Singular					
First person	I	me	my	mine	myself
Second person	you	you	your	yours	yourself
Third person	he, she, it	him, her, it	his, her, its	his, hers, its	himself herself itself
Plural					
First person	we	us	our	ours	ourselves
Second person	you	you	your	yours	yourself
Third person	they	them	their	theirs	themselves

Antecedent	The noun that is replaced by a pronoun. Pronouns must agree with their noun antecedents in three ways: number, gender, and person.
Number	Singular: *Bill* took the EKGs. He took five.
	Plural: The *doctors* gave *their* off duty time to volunteer.
Gender	Masculine singular: *Jonathan* liked *his* care.
	Feminine plural: *Medical assistants* wear *their* hair at a certain length.
Person	1st (speaker): *Norma* is my name. *I* am named after my father, Norman.
	2nd (spoken to): *Pat*, are you sure? Do you mean what you say?
	3rd (spoken about): *Norman and Leonard* know how to scrub. *They* understand surgical technique.
	Antecedents joined by *and* need a plural pronoun: *Tom and Mary* are friends. *They* study together.
	For antecedents joined by *or* or *nor*, the pronoun agrees with the nearest antecedent: Either the doctor or the *nurses* left *their* charts here.

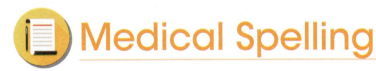

Medical Spelling

Become familiar with the spelling of the following words:

aerosols	catheter	gallbladder	palpitations
amniocentesis	cerebrovascular	glaucoma	pancreas
antibiotics	cholecystectomy	hemiplegic	pancreatitis
aneurysm	cirrhosis	hemorrhoids	paraplegia
antiemetic	coagulation	hypertension	quadriplegia
antiseptic	conjunctiva	hypotension	sphygmomanometer
auscultation	electrocardiogram	insulin	stethoscope
bronchoscopy	esophagus	meninges	urinalysis
cardiopulmonary	etiology	mesentery	
resuscitation (CPR)	fallopian tube	occlusion	
cataract	fontanel	prostatitis	

Real-World Applications

The Office Memorandum and Electronic Mail

The office memorandum or memo is a written or electronic message (email) sent to coworkers *in the same office or organization.* It is usually a short, quick message. The format may already be in your office software. Its purpose is to expedite the flow of information; ask or answer questions; describe procedures or policies; remind people of meetings or appointments; or list names, schedules, written records, pronouncements, or work activities.

They are intended for internal circulation, and they are less formal than a business letter. The writer must ensure that pronouns agree with their noun antecedents in number, gender, and person.

Writing a Memo or an Email

Some organizations have special software for office memos, but a plain piece of paper is sufficient (Figures 2-1 and 2-2). The format for the content of a memo must be very simple. Consider this structure as an example for a memo:

To:	(person to whom the message is written)
From:	(person writing the message)
Subject: (or Re:)	("secure" or "confidential" if in the medical arena, or perhaps the precise purpose or topic of the memo—ALWAYS keeping HIPAA in mind.)
Date:	(month, day, and year the memo is written)
(The message of the memo follows.)	

V
M
C

VILLES MEDICAL CENTER

OFFICE MEMO

Date: August 1, 20XX

To: Office Medical Assistants

From: Rose Villes, RN, Office Manager

Subject: Upgrade of Computer Systems

Computer World is giving a training workshop on the MedSoft Computer

Program that BMC plans to implement before September 15. Here are the details:

Tuesday, July 15, from 9 : 00 a.m. to 4 : 00 p.m.

Second Floor Conference Room

Read the enclosed brochure about the program before attending the

workshop.

C: Dr. Luke Christopher

Enc.

FIGURE 2-1 Sample Memo

In large facilities, another category may be added after the "From" line, namely, "Specialty/Floor/ Ext."

The writing style of a memo or email is direct, concise, and clear. Avoid vague messages like, "Get back to me about this matter." Replace it with, "Call me Tuesday morning, July 30." Saving an office memo or email can be very important and helpful in the medical office. In the medical office, the memo or email could contain medications or symptoms that provide information for further testing or

To:	Lorry Villes, R.N.
From:	Mary Louise Norman, M.D.
Subject:	Staff Meeting, March 5, 20XX, 9 a.m.
CC:	Louis Villes, Chairperson
Date:	February 17, 20XX

Add three additional topics to the agenda for the March 5 meeting. The topics are **as follows:**

1. Written policies regarding safety procedures
2. Documentation procedures update
3. New computer software needs

If you have any questions, call me at ext. 229.

FIGURE 2-2 An Email Format

diagnosing. It could be important for proof that something was said or done. Emails in the medical office are very confidential (please refer to HIPAA rules and laws) and should not be used when:

1. The content is highly confidential.
2. The message is long and complicated.
3. The message has the tone of being emotionally charged and could be misconstrued.
4. The email response or message has not been carefully reread and information was not checked.
5. Emails are with all upper-case or bold letters.
6. One sends an email without a name, title, phone, or extension.

Remember, even if you delete a message it can be retrieved. Always remember your audience. Emails are used frequently. Office portals are used frequently for communication. People have different opinions, and some consider the use of email unprofessional. Times are changing and emails are becoming a more convenient and easier way to communicate.

Subject lines are like newspaper headlines. They convey the main point. Please consider using the words "secure" or "confidential" in the subject line. Never, ever include anyone's social security number in an email!

Greetings and sign-offs are considerate. It is better not to start just with the text. Some common ways to address are:

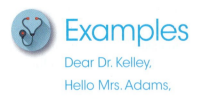

Examples

Dear Dr. Kelley,

Hello Mrs. Adams,

Hi Jacob,

If you don't know the name of the person you are addressing, here are some examples of polite generic ways to address:

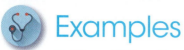

Examples

To Whom It May Concern:

Dear patient,

Dear member,

Your closing is important because it lets the reader know who you are, your title, and your office or organization. Also, for good measure, your contact number and extension may be included. For example:

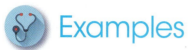

Examples

Anna Ruiz, RN, MEd

Office Manager

Offices of Dr. Trout and Villes

999-999-9999

Examples of friendly closings:

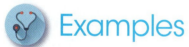

Examples

Thank you,

Best,

Regards,

And formal closings:

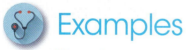

Examples

Sincerely,

Respectfully yours,

CC (carbon copy) and BCC (blind carbon copy) are ways to send your message to someone else at the same time as the person you are addressing. If you want to convey the message to another, such as the doctor you are working for and your office manager, you would use CC.

BCC (blind carbon copy) is used when you don't want everyone on the list to have each other's emails.

Additional thoughts on writing and communicating with emails:

Think about your message and do not send it in haste. What is your purpose? Who is your audience? Jot down notes and be clear when conveying your message. Put your thoughts in a logical sequence. Reread your notes or retype/rewrite your notes. Cut and paste where needed to keep the context in an orderly logical sequence. Reread: Does it say what you want to communicate? Proofread the final copy before sending. Check for spelling and grammar mistakes.

Quick questions before sending the email message:

1. What is the purpose?
2. Is this confidential and secure?
3. Is it appropriate for the audience? For the person receiving it?
4. Is it easy to read and understand?
5. Did you identify yourself?
6. Correct grammar? Correct punctuation? Are your thoughts in order?
7. Lastly, are there important items such as dates, times, and place or places highlighted?

PRACTICE 11: Memos and Email

Write an office memo that includes this information:

- change in office hours from 8 a.m. to 5 p.m. to 9 a.m. to 4 p.m.
- new hours effective only during the week between Christmas and New Year's
- applies to all staff members
- the message is from Dr. Matthews to staff members

Office Memorandum and Electronic Mail Summary

Type of Communication	Definition	Format/Structure
Memo	A written message to coworkers in the same company	**To:** **From:** **Re:** **Date:**
Email	A computer-to-computer communication system that transmits messages electronically	To: From: Subject: CC: (optional) Date:

VILLES MEDICAL CENTER

OFFICE MEMO

Date:

To:

From:

Subject:

FIGURE 2-3 Practice Office Memo

Skills Review

Circle the correct pronoun from within the parentheses:

1. Each procedure has (its, their) own requirements.

2. Lorry and (she, her) were getting the patient ready for the cholecystectomy.

3. (Who, Whom) did the cross-reference on these files?

4. The doctor appointed (he, him) to the Quality Assurance Program.

5. Someone called with a medical office emergency. I did schedule (him, them) STAT.

6. It was (she, her) who established the matrix on the appointment schedule.

7. One of the patients developed (his, their) symptoms over two years.

8. Norm and (I, me) are leaving for the conference in the morning.

9. (Who, Whom) shall we hire to do the insurance claims?

10. The PT (coagulation test) was done by (we, us).

*Circle the indefinite pronoun and above it write **S** if singular or **P** if plural:*

1. Everyone suffering from orthopnea must sit up to breathe.

2. Not one of the orthopedic patients has traction.

3. Many of our students realize that their oral communication skills are vital to their success.

4. The tumors were not visible, but he found several when he conducted the examination.

5. None of the symptoms indicated an emergency.

Circle the pronouns in the email message. Write them below and identify the type of pronoun as personal, relative, reflexive, indefinite, interrogative, or demonstrative. Identify any noun antecedents, if applicable.

EMAIL July 15, 20XX

I received your email message today. The mailing that you sent contained all laboratory reports Dr. Byrnes needed to plan his procedure. Dr. Byrnes thanks you, as does everyone here.

PRONOUN	TYPE	NOUN ANTECEDENT
_____	_____	_____
_____	_____	_____
_____	_____	_____
_____	_____	_____
_____	_____	_____
_____	_____	_____

Circle the correctly spelled word in each line:

1. coagulation	caogulation	coaguletion	coagulattion
2. antimetic	cataract	mininges	cirrhosis
3. prostetitis	prostattitis	prostatetis	Prostatitis
4. esophagus	oclusion	aerosols	anteseptic
5. hemorhoids	hemmorrhoids	hemorrhaids	hemorrhoids
6. insulin	misentery	cateter	anurysm
7. urenalysis	hypotension	cholecystectamy	meningis
8. eteology	cerebrovescular	broncuscopy	etiology
9. antibiotics	arosols	antibiautics	glowcoma
10. electrokardiogram	electrocardigram	electrocardiogram	eletrocardiogram

 # Comprehensive Review

Write an office memo to Dr. William Freeze to reschedule the August 15, 20XX meeting to August 30. Use at least three pronouns with two noun antecedents. Circle the pronouns and underline the noun antecedents. Use the format your instructor suggests.

LINCOLN MEDICAL CENTER
OFFICE MEMO

TO: DATE:

FROM:

RE:

FIGURE 2-4 Office Memo

SECTION 3
Verbs

Practical Writing Component: The Medical Record

Objectives

After reading this section, the learner should be able to:

- identify verb types
- identify transitive and intransitive verbs
- use verbs that agree with the subject
- distinguish between active and passive voices
- use principal parts of regular verbs
- use verb tenses correctly
- use the mood of verbs appropriately
- spell various medical terms
- explain the medical record/electronic health record (EHR)/electronic medical record (EMR)/medical chart
- explain AHIMA and Joint Commission
- describe the Health Insurance Portability and Accountability Act (HIPAA)

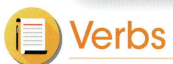 ## Verbs

The principal characteristics of a *verb* is that it expresses action or a state of being.

Action Verbs

Action verbs are words that express activity.

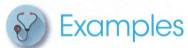

Examples

Blood *circulates* through the heart, arteries, and veins.

Ask for an appointment.

The patient *complains* of extreme thirst.

The doctor *performed* the operation.

"Being" Verbs

Verbs can also express a state of being. Any form of the verb *to be* that stands alone is a *being verb*: *am, is, are, was, were,* any form of *be* or *been.*

Examples

I *am* the nurse in charge.

Bob *is* the patient in question.

We *were* watching for obvious symptoms.

   "Being" verbs may be used as the only verb in a sentence or they may be combined with another verb. When a being verb is used with another verb, it can be a linking verb, a helping verb, or an auxiliary verb. It completes thought in words.

Examples

I *was* at the hospital.

I *was helping* the nurse.

Phil *was doing* his procedures.

The exam *was* thorough.

 PRACTICE 1: Action and Being Verbs

Identify the verb in each sentence:

1. Antibiotics are expensive. _____

2. Cataracts are common in the elderly. _____

3. Hands washed frequently prevent the transmission of disease. _____

4. Palpation is one of the five Ps. _____

5. Tetracycline® is a broad-spectrum antibiotic. _____

Main Verbs and Helping Verbs

A *helping verb* is a verb used together with the main verb for action:

Common Helping Verbs		
am	has	can (may) have
are	had	could (would, should) be
is	can	could (would, should) have
was	may	will (shall) have been
were	will (shall) be	might have
do	will (shall) have	might have been
did	has (had) been	must
have	can (may) be	must have been

The combination of a helping verb and a main verb is referred to as a verb phrase. In a verb phrase, the last verb is always the main verb.

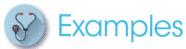 Examples

The intern *had studied* all night. [*Had* is the helping verb and *studied* is the main verb.]

Operations *were delayed* for one hour. [The verb phrase is *were delayed*.]

Verbs may be separated by other words that are not part of the verb phrase.

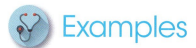 Examples

Mark *has* never *liked* working in the laboratory.

Can Dr. Villmarie *operate* next Thursday?

Linking Verbs

A *linking verb* connects the subject with a complement—a noun, pronoun, adjective, or phrase—that completes the meaning of the linking verb.

The most common linking verb is the verb *be,* which has the following forms, *am, is, are, was, were, be, being, been.* Other common linking verbs are: appear, become, feel, grow, look, seems, stay, taste, smell, remain, and sound.

Examples

Mary *is* my *assistant*. [*Is* is the linking verb; *assistant* is the complement (predicate noun).]

Luke *is* the *supervisor*. [*Is* is the linking verb; *supervisor* is the complement (noun).]

The ideas *are excellent*. [*Are* is the linking verb; *excellent* is the complement (adjective).]

 ## PRACTICE 2: Verb Phrases

Identify the verb or verb phrases in each sentence:

1. We have read the article in the journal. _____

2. A patient has the right to privacy. _____

3. Has the blood pressure been stabilized? _____

4. Fluid accumulated in the lungs. _____

5. Caffeine stimulates the nervous system. _____

Transitive and Intransitive Verbs

A *transitive verb* shows action and needs a direct object to complete its meaning.

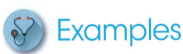 # Examples

The patient ate solid *food*. [*Food* is the *direct object*, so the verb is transitive.]

The anesthesiologist intubated the *patient*.

The surgeon sutured the *laceration*.

The surgical team changed scrub *clothes*.

Verbs that do not have a direct object are called *intransitive verbs*. These verbs have no object to receive the action.

 # Examples

The patient ate poorly. [There is no direct object, so the verb is intransitive.]

The surgeon sutured.

Cancer radiates quickly from the lymph nodes.

The students studied for three hours.

The surgical team changed.

PRACTICE 3: Transitive and Intransitive Verbs

Identify the verbs and indicate whether they are transitive or intransitive:

1. The doctor introduced the scope. _____

2. The music relaxed the surgical team in the operating room. _____

3. The intravenous catheter punctured the skin. _____

4. The trachea bifurcates into the right and left bronchi. _____

5. The test reveals normal blood cholesterol. _____

Gerunds

A *gerund* ends in *-ing* and acts as a noun.

 ## Examples

Nursing is her profession. (*Nursing* is a gerund. It acts as a noun and is the subject of the sentence.)

Dr. Tran likes *operating* at the Memorial. [*Operating* acts as a noun and is the object of the verb (direct object).]

Infinitives

An *infinitive* consists of the word *to* plus a verb. The two words together usually act as a noun.

 ## Examples

To work in the medical professions is noble. [*To work* acts as a noun and is the subject of the sentence.]

Dr. Tran likes *to operate* at the Memorial. [*To operate* acts as a noun and is the object of the verb (direct object).]

The patient was about *to speak*. [*To speak* is an infinitive; *to speak* acts as a noun and is the object of the preposition "about."]

 # Person of a Verb

Like pronouns, verbs also have first, second, and third person. Person helps determine whether the subject is singular or plural. For example:

	Singular		Plural	
1st person	I	I walk	we	we walk
2nd person	you	you walk	you	you walk
3rd person	he, she, it	he walks	they	they walk

Number of a Verb

Verbs, like nouns and pronouns, also have a number. Number indicates whether the verb is singular or plural. The verb must agree in number with the subject. If the subject is plural, the verb must be plural; if the subject is singular, the verb must be singular.

Examples

The pharmacy is conveniently located. [*Pharmacy* is singular. The verb *is* is singular.]

A *child dreams* many things when she is young.

Children dream many things when they are young.

Dr. Villmarie and *Dr. Archie operate* together.

Dr. Villmarie also *operates* alone.

Students work hard on their projects.

Valerie works harder on her anatomy than on medical terminology.

Sometimes a group of words separates the subject from the verb, but number agreement between the subject and verb must be maintained.

Examples

The *hygienists* in the office next to the garden *examine* teeth.

Terry, with the extra hours, *accumulated* vacation time.

A compound subject (two or more words joined by *and*) requires a plural verb.

Examples

The *stethoscope and reflex hammer are* tools of the physician.

Jeff and Lorry make good salaries.

When two subjects are combined by *either. . . or, neither. . . nor,* and *not only. . . but also,* the verb agrees with the subject closest to it.

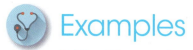 Examples

Neither Mary nor her *sister likes* to give injections.

Neither Mary nor her *sisters like* to give injections.

Not only Ernie but also his *mother lives* near the medical office.

Not only Ernie but also his *parents live* near the medical office.

 PRACTICE 4: Verb Forms

Identify the subject in each sentence and select the correct verb from within the parentheses:

1. Shock (is, are) a serious condition. _____

2. The EMTs (resuscitate, resuscitates) patients. _____

3. The instruments (need, needs) to be calibrated regularly. _____

4. The patient's tumor (has, have) impaired many systems. _____

5. Neither the physician nor the employees (disclose, discloses) patient information.
   _____

 # Verb Tenses

The English language has many *verb tenses*. This chapter covers only three: past, present, and future (Figure 3-1). These are the tenses used most frequently in the allied health setting.

Present Tense

Present tense expresses action that is happening at the *present* time, or action that happens regularly.

 Examples

You *work* in a doctor's office.

The doctor *sutures* the laceration in the ER.

The doctor *examines* the patients.

Past Tense

Past tense expresses action that was completed in the past. Notice that *-ed* is used to form the past tense of the regular verbs in the examples.

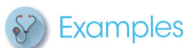

Examples

You *worked* in a doctor's office.

The doctor *sutured* the laceration in the emergency room.

The doctor *examined* the patients.

Future Tense

The *future tense* expresses action that will take place any time after the present time. To form the future tense, the word *will* is used with the main verb. *Will* is the sign of the future tense.

Examples

You *will work* in a doctor's office.

The doctor *will suture* the laceration in the emergency room.

The doctor *will examine* the patients.

	Meaning	How Formed	Examples Singular	Plural	Use in Sentence
Present	Action happens now or regularly	Use main verb	I work Your work He she, it works	We work You work They work	I work 35 hours a week now.
Past	Action begins and ends in the past	Add *d* or *ed* to the main verb	I worked You worked He, she, it workd	We workd You worked They worked	I worked 30 hours a week last year.
Future	Action will occur sometime in the future	Add *will* to the main verb	I will work You will work He, she, it will work	We will work You will work They will work	I will work 40 hours a week next year.

FIGURE 3-1 Forms of a Regular Verb

PRACTICE 5: Verb Tenses

Identify the verbs and state whether they are in the past, present, or future tense:

1. The physician decides on the most efficient scheduling policy. _____

2. The cancer originated in the lungs. _____

3. Blood cells circulate through the body in one minute. _____

4. The surgeon resected the diseased colon. _____

5. Results of the health survey will be published. _____

Principal Parts of Verbs

Verb tenses tell when an action or state of being occurs. Every verb has four principal parts for denoting tense: the present, past, past participle, and present participle. How verb forms change from one principal part to another categorizes them as regular or irregular verbs.

Regular Verbs

The past tense of regular verbs is formed by adding the letters *-d* or *-ed* to the present form of the verb. A helping verb is added to the *past* form of the verb to make a *past participle*. Adding *-ing* to the present tense forms the *present participle*.

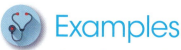 Examples

Present	Present Participle	Past	Past Participle
introduce	introducing	introduced	has, had, have introduced
look	looking	looked	has, had, have looked
tolerate	tolerating	tolerated	has, had, have tolerated
diagnose	diagnosing	diagnosed	had diagnosed
compare	comparing	compared	have compared
drop	dropping	dropped	has dropped
perform	performing	performed	has performed

Notice that some regular verbs change their spelling to form the past tense or present participle. The verb rules shown in Figures 3-2 and 3-3 help make the spelling easier.

1. Verbs ending in *e* add *d: hope, hoped.*

2. One-syllable verbs ending in a consonant preceded by one vowel double the final consonant and add *ed: stop, stopped;* preceded by two vowels add *ed: rain, rained.*

3. Two-syllable verbs ending in a consonant with the accent on the first syllable add *ed: open, opened;* with the accent on the second syllable double the final consonant and add *ed: recur, recurred.*

4. Verbs ending in two consonants add *ed: start, started.*

5. Verbs ending in *y* preceded by a vowel keep the *y* and add *ed: pray, prayed;* preceded by a consonant change *y* to *i* and *ed: try, tried.*

6. Verbs ending in *ie* add *d: lie, lied.*

FIGURE 3-2 Rules for Forming Past Tense of Regular Verbs

1. Verbs ending in *e* drop the *e* and add *ing: hope, hoping.*

2. One-syllable verbs ending in a consonant preceded by one vowel double the final consonant and add *ing: stop, stopping;* preceded by two vowels add *ing: rain, raining.*

3. Two-syllable verbs ending in a consonant with the accent on the first syllable add *ing: open, opening;* with the accent on the second syllable double the final consonant and add *ing: recur, recurring.*

4. Verbs ending in two consonants add *ing: start, starting.*

5. Verbs ending in *y* keep the *y* and add *ing: pray, praying; try, trying.*

6. Verbs ending in *ie* change the *ie* to *y* and add *ing: lie, lying.*

FIGURE 3-3 Rules for Forming the Present Participle of Regular Verbs

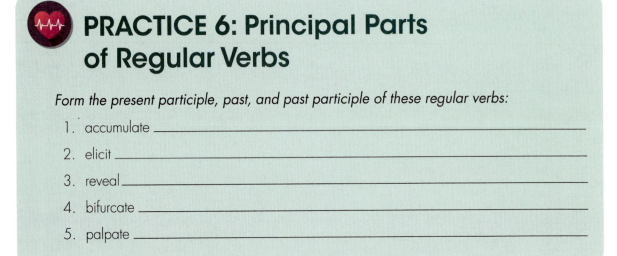

PRACTICE 6: Principal Parts of Regular Verbs

Form the present participle, past, and past participle of these regular verbs:

1. accumulate _____

2. elicit _____

3. reveal _____

4. bifurcate _____

5. palpate _____

Irregular Verbs

Only regular verbs follow the rule to add *-d* or *-ed* to form the past. Many verbs in the English language do not follow this rule. The verbs that do not are called irregular verbs.

Some irregular verbs keep the same form in three of the four parts:

Present	Present Participle	Past	Past Participle
burst	bursting	burst	had burst
cost	costing	cost	had cost
let	letting	let	had let
set	setting	set	have set
hit	hitting	hit	had hit
read	reading	read	has read
put	putting	put	had put
hurt	hurting	hurt	has hurt

Some irregular verbs change form twice:

Present	Present Participle	Past	Past Participle
sleep	sleeping	slept	had slept
say	saying	said	had said
buy	buying	bought	had bought
have	having	had	had
find	finding	found	had found

Some irregular verbs change three forms:

Present	Present Participle	Past	Past Participle
eat	eating	ate	had eaten
tear	tearing	tore	had torn
throw	throwing	threw	had thrown
break	breaking	broke	had broken
drink	drinking	drank	had drunk
forgive	forgiving	forgave	had forgiven

Many errors are made using irregular verbs. Try to memorize as many principal parts of irregular verbs as possible. See Table 3-1 for the more commonly encountered irregular verb forms.

TABLE 3-1 Past and Past Participle Forms of Common Irregular Verbs

Simple Present	Past	Past Participle	Simple Present	Past	Past Participle
awake	awoke	awoken	know	knew	known
am/are	was/were	been	leave	left	left
beat	beat	beaten	lose	lost	lost
begin	began	begun	make	made	made
bend	bent	bent	prove	proved	proven
bite	bit	bitten	ring	rang	rung
blow	blew	blown	run	ran	run
bring	brought	brought	see	saw	seen
burst	burst	burst	send	sent	sent
catch	caught	caught	sew	sewed	sewn
choose	chose	chosen	shake	shook	shaken
come	came	come	show	showed	shown
cost	cost	cost	shut	shut	shut
cut	cut	cut	sing	sang	sung
do	did	done	sit	sat	sat
draw	drew	drawn	slay	slew	slain
drive	drove	driven	slit	slit	slit
fall	fell	fallen	speak	spoke	spoken
feed	fed	fed	spread	spread	spread
fight	fought	fought	spring	sprang	sprung
flee	fled	fled	steal	stole	stolen
fly	flew	flown	strive	strove	striven
find	found	found	swell	swelled	swollen
forget	forgot	forgotten	swim	swam	swum
freeze	froze	frozen	take	took	taken
get	got	gotten	tear	tore	torn
give	gave	given	throw	threw	thrown
go	went	gone	wake	woke	woken
grow	grew	grown	wear	wore	worn
hang	hung	hung	wring	wrung	wrung
hide	hid	hidden	write	wrote	written
hold	held	held			

 # PRACTICE 7: Irregular Verbs

Select the correct verb form from within the parentheses:

1. The movement (elicit, elicited) the symptoms.

2. I had (spoke, spoken) to the nurse about the change.

3. The symptoms (occur, occurred) as a result of inadequate circulation.

4. The driver had (drive, drove, driven) the ambulance right up to the door.

5. The nurse (shook, shake, shaken) the bottle to mix the medication.

Confusing and Troublesome Verbs

Some verbs are frequently confused with verbs that seem to mean the same thing. Even coming up with the correct forms for their principal parts can be troublesome. Errors are made frequently with these verbs, both orally and written. A brief explanation of some troublesome verbs may be helpful.

Lie and *Lay*

Lie means "recline, rest, or stay," as in "I need to *lie* down for a while." *Lay* means "put or place," as in "*Lay* your head on the pillow." Here are the principal parts of those two verbs:

Present	Past	Past Participle	Present Participle
lie	lay	lain	lying (reclining)
lay	laid	laid	laying (placing)

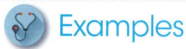 Examples

I *lay* the book on the table.

I *lie* down.

I *lay* down yesterday.

I *have lain* down.

PRACTICE 8: Lie and Lay

Fill in the correct form of the verb lie or lay and state whether the action is to recline or to place:

1. She has _____ in bed all day. _____

2. The sick patient _____ ill for days. _____

3. The M.A. had _____ the instruments out for the procedure. _____

4. Where did I _____ my lab coat? _____

5. The medications were _____ on the table. _____

Rise and *Raise*

Rise means "to move upward by itself or to get up," as in "Temperatures *rise* in the afternoon." *Raise* means "to lift to a higher position," as in "*Raise* the cost of medicine by 2 percent." Here are the principal parts of these two verbs:

Present	Present Participle	Past	Past Participle
rise	rising	rose	has risen
raise	raising	raised	had raised

Examples

We *raised* the treatment table an inch higher.

Medical costs *rise*.

Costs *rose* frequently last year.

Costs have *risen*.

 # PRACTICE 9: Rise and Raise

Fill in the correct form of the verbs rise or raise: State whether the action is to lift to a higher position, to move upward by itself or to get up.

1. Did the patient's diet _____ the blood chemistry levels?

2. The potassium has _____ to normal levels.

3. The patient did not _____ enough sputum for the test.

4. Elevated cholesterol in the blood _____ the risk of coronary disease.

5. They _____ the level of medication needed for the test.

The key distinction between *lie/lay* and *rise/raise* is that *lay* and *raise* are transitive (the sentence has a direct object) and *lie* and *rise* are intransitive (the sentence has no object).

May and Can

Errors are often made between the words *may* and *can*. *May* means permission or a degree of certainty. To use the word *may* is considered polite.

 ## Examples

You *may* leave at 4:30 p.m. [permission]

May I please borrow your stethoscope? [permission]

The report *may* be true. [degree of certainty]

Can means an ability or a possibility because certain conditions exist.

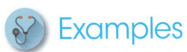 ## Examples

You *can* see the pain in her face. [ability]

A puncture wound *can* cause tetanus. [ability]

I *can* perform the procedure if I get back on time. [possibility]

PRACTICE 10: May and Can

Select the correct word from within the parentheses:

1. Call me if you think I (can, may) be of any help.
2. The nurse (can, may) perform that type of procedure.
3. The decision (may, can) determine the patient's quality of life.
4. You (may, can) be familiar with the characteristics of the disease.
5. I (may, can) work on the lab report if you (can, may) find the statistical data.

Use of Verb Tenses in Sentences

Verb tenses express the time of action. Errors arise when the time elements in different parts of a sentence do not agree. For example, the use of verb tense in the following sentence is incorrect:

When we *are tired,* we *rested* at the hotel.

The sentence starts in the present tense, *when we are tired,* but according to the rest of the sentence the present action is complete in the past, *we rested at the hotel.* An action begun in the present cannot be completed in the past because it is still occurring. The sentence should read:

When we *are tired,* we *rest* at the hotel.

Similarly:

When Valerie *was* young, she likes to *visit* her grandmother. [incorrect]
When Valerie *was* young, she *liked* to *visit* her grandmother. [correct]

PRACTICE 11: Verb Tense

Correct the verb tenses in these sentences:

1. The doctor will read the chart before he saw the patient. _____
2. If she is smart, she asked for a consultation. _____
3. Time flew quickly while we had cleaned the storage closet. _____
4. I would schedule an appointment if I have better insurance. _____
5. Aseptic hand washing is crucial if we wanted to prevent transmission of pathogens.
   _____

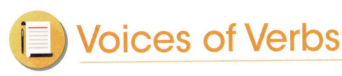

Voices of Verbs

The *voices of verbs* show whether the subject of the verb is doing the action (active) or receiving the action (passive).

Active and Passive Verbs

Verbs have two voices: active and passive. If the subject is doing the action, the verb is in the active voice. If the subject is receiving the action, the verb is in the passive voice.

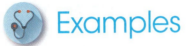 Examples

Example	Voice	Explanation
Bob mailed the letter.	Active	*Bob,* the subject of the sentence, performs the action of the verb, *mailed.* The subject, *Bob,* is busy and *actively* in motion.
The letter was mailed by Bob.	Passive	The subject, *letter,* is the receiver of the action of the verb, *mailed.* The subject of the sentence *passively* receives the action.

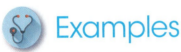 Examples

Ken typed three reports a day. [active]

　Three reports were typed by Ken. [passive]

The doctor disclosed the information. [active]

　The information was disclosed by the doctor. [passive]

The students transmitted the disease. [active]

　The disease was transmitted by the students. [passive]

The surgeon resected the tumor. [active]

　The tumor was resected by the surgeon. [passive]

Compare the active and passive voices in the previous sentences. Which voice is heard more often when people speak? Which voice seems easier to speak and understand? Most grammarians agree that the active voice is easier to understand and has more energy. The active voice quickly tells who did what, not what was done by whom. Writers who use the grammar check on the computer will note that the use of the passive voice is discouraged. However, some grammarians feel that because the passive voice is grammatically correct, it has a place in the English language. The following example shows how the passive voice may simplify a sentence.

| Active | Someone on the ethics committee made the decision on October 15. |
| Passive | The decision *was made* on October 15. |

The words *someone on the ethics committee* are not necessary to the meaning of the sentence, unless the name of the actor is specifically requested.

The Passive Voice

Two elements help detect the passive voice: (1) a being verb and (2) a past participle. Another signal is the frequent appearance of the word *by* in sentences using the passive voice.

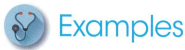 Examples

Three reports a day *were* [being verb] *typed* [past participle] *by* Ken.

The information *was* [being verb] *disclosed* [past participle] *by* the doctor.

The disease *was* [being verb] *transmitted* [past participle] *by* the students.

Water *was drunk by* the thirsty patients.

The passive voice can be changed to the active voice simply by making the direct object the subject. In the passive sentence "Water was drunk by the *patients*," the direct object is *patients*. Make it the subject of the sentence to achieve active voice: *"Patients* drank the water."

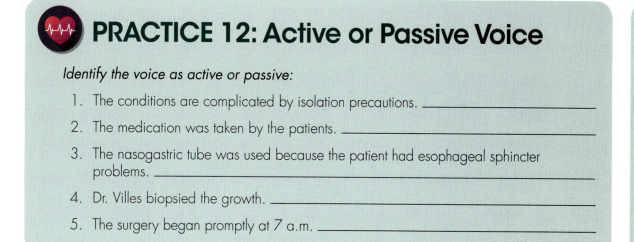

PRACTICE 12: Active or Passive Voice

Identify the voice as active or passive:

1. The conditions are complicated by isolation precautions. _____

2. The medication was taken by the patients. _____

3. The nasogastric tube was used because the patient had esophageal sphincter problems. _____

4. Dr. Villes biopsied the growth. _____

5. The surgery began promptly at 7 a.m. _____

PRACTICE 12: Active or Passive Voice

Moods of Verbs

Mood is the manner in which the action of the sentence is performed. Mood depends on the attitude of the speaker or writer and the purpose of the sentence. Verbs have three moods: indicative, imperative, and subjunctive.

The purpose of the indicative mood is to state a fact or ask a question.

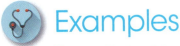 Examples

The medical assistant types reports.

The medical assistant admits the patient.

The purpose of the imperative mood is to give instruction or commands, or to make requests. The subject of verbs in the imperative mood is always *you,* the person to whom the order is given. The *you* is often omitted from the sentence.

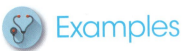 Examples

Type this report.

Take the vital signs.

The purpose of the subjunctive mood is to express a command, preference, strong request, or a condition contrary to fact. The present subjunctive is formed in two ways: (1) by substituting *be* in place of *am, are,* or *is* and (2) by dropping the *s* ending from the third person singular, present tense verb. The past subjunctive is the same as the past tense except that the verb *be* uses *were* for both singular and plural subjects.

 Examples

The doctor requests that her report *be* typed within 24 hours.

The medical assistant wished she *were* able to type the report within 24 hours.

 PRACTICE 13: Mood of Verbs

Indicate whether the verbs are in the indicative, imperative, or subjunctive mood:

1. We urge that the doctor be given a second chance. _____

2. Heart disease is the leading cause of death. _____

3. Please remove the soiled linens immediately. _____

4. The cardiologist insisted that the EKG be done again. _____

5. Tell the people in the lab that the blood tests must be done today.

_____

Verbs Summary

Types of Verbs

Action verb	Expresses both physical and mental activity.	The doctor *operates* on patients. The patient *thought* he was in good health.
Being verb	Any form of the verb to be: *am, is, are, was, were, be, being, been.*	Erythromycin *is* the cure for bacterial pneumonia.
Main verb	A single verb in a sentence.	The x-ray *revealed* a fracture in the arm.
Helping verb	A verb that accompanies the main verb: *do, will, would, can, could, shall, should, may, might, must, have, has, had.*	The x-ray *may reveal* a fracture. Many *do believe* that disease is curable.
Linking verb	Connects a complement (predicate noun, pronoun, adjective).	The students *felt comfortable* about the changes.
	Common linking verbs: *being verbs, grow, seem, appear, stay, taste.*	The patient *appears* self-motivated. The diet *seems* well planned.
Transitive verb	Shows action and needs an object to complete its meaning.	You must remove the *sutures.*
Intransitive verb	A verb that has no object to receive the action.	The medical report is filed.
Gerund	Verb + *ing;* acts as a noun	The doctor is *operating.*
Infinitive	*To* + verb; acts as a noun, verb, adjective, or adverb.	The doctor wants *to operate.*
Person of a verb	Person speaking (first).	*I* love my medical terminology course. (singular)
	Person spoken to (second).	Do *you* need more medication? (singular or plural)
	Person spoken about (third).	*They* formed an ethics team. (plural)
Number of verb	Indicates singular or plural.	He *arrives* at the ER. (singular verb agrees with singular pronoun)

Verb Tenses

Present	Action happening now.	The nurse works now.
Past	Action completed in the past.	The nurse worked yesterday.
Future	Action will happen later.	The nurse will work tomorrow.

See chapter figures for explanation of additional tenses.

Principal Parts of Speech Regular:

Past	Forms the past by adding *e* or *ed* to the *present* form of the verb (cure + d = cured).	The doctor *cured* the patient.
Past participle	Add a *helping verb* to form the *past* form (had + cured = had cured).	The doctor *had cured* the patient.
Present participle	Add *ing* to the *present* form of the verb (cure + ing = curing).	The medicine is *curing* the patient.

Irregular:

Past	came	The message *came* by telephone.
Past participle	had come	He *had come* to the end of the paragraph.
Present participle	coming	I'm *coming* to that conclusion.

Voices of Verbs:	Shows whether the subject does the action or receives the action.	
Active	The subject does the actions.	The *doctor* made the incision.
Passive	The subject receives the action.	The *incision* was made by the doctor.

Moods of Verbs	The manner in which verbs are expressed.	
Indicative	States a fact or asks a question.	Medical examinations are expensive.
Imperative	Makes a request, gives a command or instruction (subject is always the word you).	(you) Take these instruments and sterilize them.
Subjunctive	Expresses a command, preference, strong request, or condition contrary to fact.	The patient insists that all other treatments be exhausted before undergoing chemotherapy.

Medical Spelling

Become familiar with the spelling of the following words:

accompany	irrigate	deteriorate	resuscitate
accumulate	ligate	deviate	reveal
administer	occur, occurred,	disclose	stabilize
bifurcate	occurrence	elicit	sterilize
calibrate	originate	evaluate	stimulate
circulate	operate	examine	suture
complicate	palpate	radiate	tolerate
complain	perform	recur, recurred,	puncture
incubate	pulsate	recurrence	
introduce	compose	refer	
intubate	diagnose	resect	

Real-World Applications

The skills of effectively using nouns, pronouns, and verbs are necessary in all types of medical writing. The medical record is one example of medical writing that requires concise sentences with clear subject-verb agreement, as it is written proof that a procedure was done or medicine given. Data gathered from medical records are used for diagnosing and assessing a patient's condition.

The Medical Record

Health care workers and medical assistants are on the front line of the changes in the privacy of the medical health record. It is important for all of us in the medical field to understand the involvement and evolution of this crucial part of health care.

The *medical record*—also known as medical charts, health records, electronic health records, and electronic medical records (EMR)—describes and documents the history of a person's health care. It is a conglomeration and accumulation of a person's medical history. The purpose of this is to use the information within the record to give informed patient care and planning. Traditionally speaking the record contains progress notes, nurse's notes, procedures, any operative notes, radiology reports, ob-gyn notes, admission notes, discharge notes, pathology reports, history and physical notes, and test results, to name a few. It provides a basis for planning patient care. It is used for payment plans and insurance providers. It is a legal record providing evidence that the patient has received that particular care; be it medications, procedures, and/or other vital information. It is a chronological record of landmarks in a patient's health history.

Some physicians and health facilities keep the medical health record for an indefinite period of time. Remember the physician or the facility owns the physical record itself. However, the patient owns the information in the medical record. For this reason, health personnel are responsible for safeguarding the confidentiality of the patient. Many employees are required to sign a confidentiality statement.

Laws and regulations govern the disclosure of medical records.

The American Health Information Management Association

In 1928, the American College of Surgeons wanted to elevate and progress the standards of clinical health records. This led to the establishment of the Association of Record Librarians of North America (ARLNA). ARLNA wanted the health care records of hospitals and other health institutions to have better standards. In 1938, ARLNA became the American Association of Medical Records Librarians (AAMRL). In the 1960s, Medicare, Medicaid, and computers were introduced into health care. As a result of these changes, AAMRL changed its name again, this time to the American Medical Record Association (AMRA). AMRA was founded in 1970 to improve the standards of documentation, but also those of health care. In the early days of medical documentation, the patient's record consisted of a variety of "notes" or "notations" that gave very little information. Today, the medical record is a complex file of multiform documents.

Technological growth came at a very fast pace in the 1980s and 1990s. In 1991, the American Medical Records Association changed its name again to American Health Information Management Association, or AHIMA. Since the 1990s there has been incredible growth in the technology of medical health records and the advancement of HIPAA and patient confidentiality.

Due to the growth of medical technology and the need to adhere to HIPAA laws, the health industry recognizes AHIMA as the leader in governing health information management. The mission of AHIMA is to promote the best practices and standards for the health information management community. AHIMA is working to progress and implement the advancement of the electronic health records/electronic medical records.

Joint Commission

In order to achieve accreditation in health care facilities, the medical health record must comply with correctness and quality standards. Because health care workers and medical assistants deal frequently with the health care records/medical records/paperless EHR/EMR, it is important to understand that the medical record is part of the accreditation process in the health care setting.

In 1951, the Joint Commission on Accreditation of Hospitals was created, combining the programs run by the American Hospital Association, the American College of Physicians, and the American Medical Association with those of the Canadian Medical Association. It was to promote hospital reforms and management of patient care. In 1987, it was renamed the Joint Commission on Accreditation of Healthcare Organizations (JCAHO) to reflect its responsibility for accrediting all health care facilities.

In 2007, as a result of more major changes, JCAHO was renamed again; it became known simply as the *Joint Commission*. This change made the name easier to remember. One of the Joint Commission's responsibilities, again, is to accredit health care organizations and institutions.

In order to achieve accreditation status, a facility's medical records must meet certain standards regarding entries, types of information documented, formats, correction procedures, completeness of data, timely recordings, dates, signatures, and various legal documents.

As you continue in your medical career, consider these important points for well-documented medical health records:

1. Use short accurate phrases and sentences.

2. If there is a space left blank, draw a line through it so no one can write or type in the space.

3. Proofread all entries.

4. Never use correction fluid.

5. Never document before the fact.

6. Use only approved abbreviations.

7. Be absolutely sure you have the correct chart before writing.

8. State facts.

9. Record the date and time of entry.

❤ PRACTICE 14: Medical Records

Respond to these items:

1. State three purposes for the medical record.

   _____

   _____

   _____

2. Name four items found in the medical record.

   _____

   _____

   _____

   _____

3. What is the meaning of Joint Commission?

   _____

4. Who owns the information in the medical record?

   _____

5. Documenting and charting includes all of the following except _____

    a. patient's reaction to procedures   c. insurance bills

    b. medications   d. tests

Answer true or false to these statements:

1. Opinions may be added to the medical record. _____

2. The American Medical Association (AMA) provides accreditation to medical facilities. _____

3. The medical record is a legal document. _____

4. Sentences but not phrases are used in the medical record. _____

The Health Insurance Portability and Accountability Act of 1996

The *Health Insurance Portability and Accountability Act of 1996 (HIPAA)* mandates regulation and control of medical records. Organizations have had to increase privacy with the computerized medical record. The efficiency and standards vary from state to state. They differ in their enactment, governing, and regulating their own laws when it comes to the disclosure of health information. The date established by HIPAA for health care providers to implement and comply with HIPAA regulations was April 14, 2003. The Department of Health and Human Services (DHHS) at the Office for Civil Rights is authorized to enforce these regulations. Much has transpired since its inception. Many regulations govern the privacy of patients' information. It is important to stress that individuals have the right to access their own records. When HIPAA was instituted it was meant that an individual could take their insurance (portability) from one employer to another without having a preexisting condition. It also included provisions to fight against industry fraud. It included points about moving on to electronic records, EHRs. This prompted further privacy and security rules. New compliance regulations for EHRs came in 2009 with the Health Information Technology for Economic and Clinical Health Act (HITECH). Privacy regulations for health-related businesses were spelled out in 2013 since the largest breaches in the HIPAA were with health-related businesses. This act sets how health information is used and gives the patient greater access and control over their personal information and how it is used by their providers and health plans. Consequences of misuse of private information can result in criminal penalties.

Protecting patients' privacy and confidentiality regarding health care information is a critical issue in all health care environments.

Protected Health Information (PHI) in electronic form has two sets of requirements:

1. HIPAA Privacy Rule—guidelines to confidentiality

2. HIPAA Security Rule—National standards to protect electronic data that is created, received, maintained, or transmitted.

Over 91,000 violations were reported between 2003 and 2013. There were 22,000 enforcement actions and 521 were referred to the U.S. Department of Justice for criminal investigation.

HIPAA violations can be as small as discussing a patient's private health information at dinner with another health care worker. It can be meeting in an elevator to discuss the patient's health care. Violations and failures to implement HIPAA regulations can result in fines ranging from $100 to $250,000 and/or imprisonment.

The U.S. Department of Health and Human Services has investigated many cases that needed compliance. Complaints have been against pharmacies, major health centers, insurance groups, hospital chains, and small providers. The following lists some of the issues that have been reported:

1. Misuse and disclosure of Protected Health Information (PHI)
2. No protection in place of health information
3. Patients unable to access their health information
4. Using more than necessary of the protected health information
5. No safeguards of the electronic protected health information

(HS.gov/enforcement, 2013)

Some important points for health care students:

- Many regulations and laws govern the privacy of patient information, but it is important to stress that patients have the right to access their own records.

- Health professionals are obligated to protect any information of a patient that needs to be disposed.

- Discussion about patients are prohibited outside the medical setting, within any public area of the health facility, or beyond workday hours.

- Many types of information, both personal and medical, comprise the identity of a patient. Examples of medical information are found in written documents, materials sent by fax or email, words spoken by patients, or data stored in a computer. All personal information that identifies a patient, such as a social security number and medical record number, must be secured and protected. Health professionals are obligated to protect any information that needs to be disposed of, either by locking it in shredding bins or placing it directly into the shredder.

- Health care facilities that initially treat patients need to know specific health information that is essential to the care of the patient. However, caution is required about sharing patient information among other health care personnel. The disclosure of information needs to be limited to the minimum amount necessary to accomplish its purpose.

- Once a patient has left the unit, there is no need to share health information about that patient, nor is there any need for initial caregivers to know subsequent health information. If the caregiver has continued interest in the patient, the caregiver may ask the patient how he or she is feeling.

- Discussions about patients are prohibited outside the medical setting, within any public area of the health facility, or beyond workday hours. Curtains should be closed to protect a patient's physical privacy from visitors or other patients who pass through the unit or clinic.

 ## PRACTICE 15: Regulations of Medical Records

Answer true or false to the following statements:

1. HIPAA is strictly for nurses in the medical profession. _____

2. HIPAA was implemented in 1996. _____

3. Anyone who signs a release form has access to a patient's information. _____

4. One objective of HIPAA is to reduce health care fraud and abuse. _____

5. The advancement of technology has set the stage for potential violation of privacy. _____

6. HITECH is a computer company. _____

7. HIPAA and TJC are the same organization. _____

8. It is okay to talk about the patient's diagnosis to the medical secretary in the office. _____

 # Skills Review

Following the completed example given as item 1, fill in the missing part of each verb. In the fourth column, state whether the verb is regular or irregular.

Present Tense	Past Tense	Past Participle	Regular/Irregular
1. write	wrote	was written	irregular
2. operate		was operated	
3.	ran	have run	
4. see	saw	had seen	
5. go		have gone	
6. fall			
7.	cared		
8.		have diagnosed	
9. take	took		
10.	dictated		

Identify the verbs in the following sentences as transitive or intransitive:

1. The doctor hired an attorney to settle the claim. _____

2. The lawyer arrived late for the meeting. _____

3. The judge appeared impatient. _____

4. The lawyer presented his case to the judge. _____

5. The judge ruled in favor of the patient. _____

Circle the verb phrase in each sentence:

1. The decision was made.

2. By the end of this year, the book will have been printed.

3. Each new employee is required to have a physical exam.

4. Many patients are fearful and tense.

5. Hypertension has been called the silent disease.

Circle the correct verb from within the parentheses:

1. Everyone in the hospital (know, knows) Judy is the best nurse.

2. Patients (appreciate, appreciates) good health care.

3. When I went to the hospital, I was (took, take, taken) to the emergency room.

4. The problem (is, are) we have no empty beds.

5. A young or older person (make, makes) choices in life.

Simplify these sentences correctly:

1. Sutures came in a variety of materials such as silk and catgut which is from sheep's intestines. _____

2. The type of sutures which the surgeon ties each stitch separately is called interrupted. _____

3. The diameter (gauge) of the suture material vary from fine (11–0) to very coarse (3). _____

4. The 6-0 suture is also called six aught and might be wrote 000000. It is very fine. _____

5. Whole numbers such as 1, 2, 3, and 4 imply that the suture is very large diameter thread. This is very coarse suture material. _____

Answer true or false to the following:

1. A medical record can never be used for research on certain diseases.
    _____

2. Attorneys may use the medical record for litigation purposes. _____

3. Any type of abbreviations and symbols may be used in the medical record.
    _____

4. Information in the medical report is available for anyone who needs it.
    _____

5. If an activity isn't recorded in the medical documentation, it didn't happen.
    _____

6. Physicians may keep medical records forever. _____

7. One example of information found in the medical record is chemistry reports.
    _____

Circle the correct spelling in each line:

1. punchered   resucitate   sterilised   radiate
2. biforcate   pulsat   stabilised   irrigate
3. reconect   irigate   examine   operatted
4. transmitted   transmited   transmmitted   transmiited
5. incubatte   circulate   refferred   imapairr
6. diviate   deveate   deviate   deviatte
7. acompanied   accompannied   acomppanied   accompanied
8. vomet   originate   irigate   reconect
9. diteriorate   detteriorate   deteriorate   detereorat
10. examine   acumulate   administir   desclose

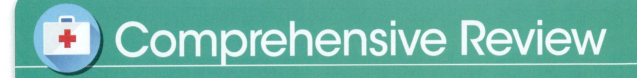

Comprehensive Review

Circle the correct word from within the parenthesis:

First impressions are lasting impressions. Health care professionals help (project, projects) a positive image to all people (who, whom) they encounter in the medical environment. Medical assistants with a good appearance (has, have) an effect on the patients they (meet, met) daily. The impression that a medical assistant (portrays, portray) to the patients (color, colors) the image of the physician and the care the patients expect.

Good grooming is essential in fostering good impressions. Good grooming (include, includes) a bath or shower daily, use of deodorant, and good oral hygiene. Hair should be (clean, cleaned), neatly styled, and above the collar. Shoes should be comfortable. Laces in shoes (need, needs) to be washed often.

The usual attire in the medical setting (is, are) uniforms, depending on the dress code of the medical facility. A uniform (give, gives) the impression of professionalism and (identify, identifies) the person as a member of the health care team. Wear a clean uniform to work daily. In offices where a uniform is not (required, requires), the medical assistant is expected to show good taste in selecting and wearing a professional wardrobe.

The amount of jewelry (is, are) limited to an engagement ring, wedding band, or professional pin. Sometimes staff members (wear, wears) name tags to help patients (identify, identifies) the health care provider by name.

A frequent problem that (surface, surfaces) with health care workers (is, are) burnout. Medical assistants need to take care of (himself, herself, themselves). Good health habits (include, includes) frequent exercise, eight hours of sleep each night, and eating the right kinds of food.

Good appearance and good health habits (is, are) important habits to foster in health care professionals.

Write the correct word above the incorrect italicized word:

The law maintains that each physician is responsible for their own negligence when someone is injured. A physician is also responsible for the negligent act performs by medical assistant employed in their office. An injured party generally sue the doctor because there is a better chance of collecting more money. A medical assistant is not licensed to practice medicine. One must be careful what he or she discuss with the patient. Patients may think the medical assistants remarks are those of the physician. These facts illustrates the importance of performing all actions with extreme care.

Select the BEST answer that identifies the underlined words in each sentence:

1. *Charting* and *documenting* are instruments that hold the medical team accountable for services rendered to patients.

   a. infinitive   b. gerunds   c. linking verbs   d. helping verbs

2. Data obtained from the medical record *does* help in the treatment of patients.

   a. action verb   b. intransitive verb   c. being verb   d. helping verb

3. Scientists *had found* critical evidence regarding medications and test results.

   a. present tense   b. past tense   c. past participle   d. present participle

4. A cohesive method is needed *to give* information to physicians and supportive staff.

   a. gerund   b. infinitive   c. linking verb   d. present participle.

5. Health care facilities *must follow* HIPAA standards for faxing health care information.

   a. imperative   b. indicative   c. subjunctive   d. none of these answers

SECTION 4
Adjectives

Practical Writing Component: Reports

Adjectives

Three important parts of speech have been explained—nouns, pronouns, and verbs. These words are important because the noun (or pronoun, which takes the place of a noun) and verb constitute the main part of a sentence. A sentence must have a noun or pronoun (*you*) as the subject and a verb in order to express a complete thought; otherwise, there is no sentence. However, additional words or parts of speech are used to make sentences clearer and more enjoyable to read and write. These additional words—adjectives and adverbs—complement, describe, add meaning to, or explain the noun and verb (Figure 4-1).

This chapter explains the part of speech called an adjective. An *adjective* is a word that describes a noun or pronoun. It adds to the meaning of the noun or pronoun by giving more information about it. In the sentences that follow, notice how the adjectives further clarify the nouns they modify:

The *new* members of the team will arrive next week.

The doctor gives a *thorough* examination.

Noun	Verb	Additional Clarifying Words
Nurses	observe	Nurses observe *reactions to treatments.*
Doctors	operate	Doctors operate in *emergency situations.*
He	speaks	He speaks *with authority about accreditation.*
MAs	transcribe	MAs transcribe *medical reports*

FIGURE 4-1 Adding Meaning to Sentences

Hospital policies often require *legal* consultation.

These grades show knowledge of *body* systems.

Your *license* renewal is due *this* month.

Limiting Adjectives

Adjectives describe four important facts about nouns and pronouns by answering the questions *which one? how many? how much?* and *what kind?* Adjectives that answer the first three questions are called *limiting adjectives* because they limit the nouns to a definite or indefinite amount. Common limiting adjectives are *a, an, all, any, both, each, every, few, many, more, most, much, no, some, such, this, that, these, those, the, one* (or any other number), and *possessive nouns* and *pronouns* used as adjectives.

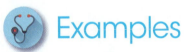 Examples

some diseases	*two* patients	*this* streptococcal
many meetings	*each* day	*the* myocardial infarction
a necrotic tumor	*an* exam	*my* medication
our office	*your* license	*their* medical records

All pathological findings should be recorded.

These charts are going to the Medical Records Department.

Their system works best for that individual practice.

A and AN

A and *an* are limiting adjectives called *indefinite articles.* When deciding between the use of *a* or *an*, consider the sound of the word that follows the article rather than its spelling. The *a* is used before words that begin with a consonant sound, a long *u* (as in "university"), and an *o* with the sound of a *w* (as in "one"). The *an* is used before words that begin with all other vowel sounds. *The* is a limiting adjective called a definite article.

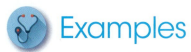

a uric acid test	*a* cross section	*an* inguinal hernia
an unsuccessful medication	*an* antidiuretic pill	*an* asset
an honor	*a* uniform	*an* eight-hour day
an abdominal incision		

Singular and Plural

A limiting adjective must agree with the noun or pronoun it limits. Limiting adjectives used with singular nouns are *a, an, each, every, either, this, that, neither,* and *one.*

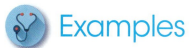

an order	*either* instrument	*neither* doctor	*one* calculus
every patient	*this* bed	*every* report	*each* stitch

Limiting adjectives used with plural nouns are *few, several, many, these, those,* and *two* (or any number other than one).

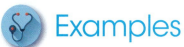

These reports need to be filed tomorrow.

Several reports must be transcribed by tomorrow morning.

The limiting adjectives *all, any,* and *some* can be either singular or plural.

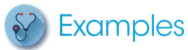

all data   *some* information   *any* problems

Some limiting adjectives may change into other parts of speech, depending on how they are used in a sentence. One example is the adjective *many,* which can be used as an adjective or a pronoun. If the word modifies a noun or pronoun, it is an adjective. If the word functions alone as a subject, direct object, indirect object, or object of a preposition, it is a pronoun.

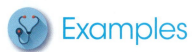

Limiting Adjective	*Many* medical assistants are taking the certification exam. [*Many* describes the noun *assistants* and is used as an adjective.]
Pronoun	*Many* of the medical assistants are taking the certification exam. [*Many* is used alone as a subject pronoun.]

Interrogative and Proper Adjectives

Two limiting adjectives, *which* and *what,* are called *interrogative adjectives* because they ask *direct* or *indirect* questions. In the first case, a question is asked directly by the person wanting the answer. An additional step is added with the *indirect* question. The question is asked for someone else. *Which* is used when the speaker wants someone to make a choice among alternatives.

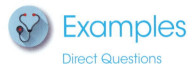 Examples

Direct Questions	*What* time is it, Bill?
	Which room is available for the patient?
Indirect Questions	The nurse wants to know *which* hours she will be working.
	The nurse wants to know *what* time the doctor is expected.

A *proper adjective* has its source within a proper noun, such as the word *Italian,* which comes from the proper noun *Italy.* Like the proper noun, the proper adjective begins with a capital letter.

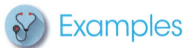 Examples

Italian spaghetti   *Spanish* influence   *American* citizen

Eponyms are also proper adjectives. An eponym comes from the surname of a person after which something is named, as in *Foley* catheter or *Mayo* scissors. (Because eponyms are important in medical documentation, more information is provided in a separate section later in this chapter.)

Predicate and Compound Adjectives

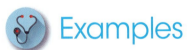 Examples

Smoking is *dangerous* to your health. [*Dangerous* is in the predicate, follows the linking verb *is,* and describes the noun *smoking.*]

Health fairs are *educational.*

Adjectives may also be used as predicate adjectives. Like their noun counterparts, *predicate adjectives* come after *linking* verbs.

The word "compound" means to combine two or more elements. *Compound adjectives* combine two or more describing words that act as a single describer. When the compound adjective comes before the noun it describes, it is usually hyphenated for clarity. When the compound adjective comes after the noun it describes, a hyphen is not usually used.

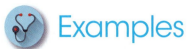

Examples

The hospital has *state-of-the-art* technology. [before the noun]

The technology at the hospital is *state of the art*. [after the noun]

She had *second-degree* burns on her upper extremities. [before]

The burns on her upper extremities were *second degree*. [after]

A number plus a noun of single measurement (*16-unit*) is hyphenated when it comes before the noun. The number and noun are not hyphenated when they follow a noun.

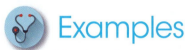

Examples

The hospital is a *six-story* building.	The hospital has *six stories*.
The *one-inch* wound needed sutures.	The wound with sutures was *one inch*.

Fractions are hyphenated when they are spelled out.

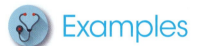

Examples

two-thirds, one-half   *Two-thirds* of the faculty were women.

Some frequently used adjectives are not hyphenated because they are considered one word.

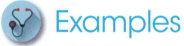

Examples

childbirth   earache   nosebleed   painless

In a series of adjectives with the same root word, omit all but the last root word.

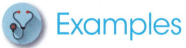

Examples

Incorrect	The medicine will take *5-bottle, 10-bottle,* and *12-bottle* sizes.
Correct	The medicine will take 5-, 10-, and *12-bottle* sizes.
Correct	The report will have a four- to *six-week* delay.

A comma is placed between two or more adjectives that express different concepts about the noun they describe.

PRACTICE 1: Adjectives

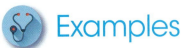 Examples

The *young, polite* intern expressed good bedside manners.

The ambulance was a *large, colorful* vehicle.

The ambulance was a *large, well-equipped* vehicle.

 PRACTICE 1: Adjectives

Choose the correct limiting adjective from within the parentheses:

1. (Many, A) nurse works on the third floor.

2. (A, An) nurse likes to work on the first shift.

3. (One, Two) elevators are available for ambulatory patients.

4. The doctor ordered (these, this) medications a week ago.

5. (Several, Each) alarm goes off when the emergency door is opened.

Hyphenate the adjectives where necessary:

1. The laboratory uses state of the art technology.

2. The doctor made many off the record comments.

3. Katy's medical record is up to date.

4. Ready to wear uniforms are popular with nurses.

5. A well known physician will do the operation.

Descriptive Adjectives

Descriptive adjectives modify nouns or pronouns by describing their characteristics or qualities. Descriptive adjectives are perhaps the easiest type of adjective to understand. They provide clarity by adding specifics about the nouns they describe. Adjectives that tell *what kind* are called descriptive adjectives.

 Examples

The *tall* nurse wore a *white* uniform.

The *streptococcal* infection spread through the *respiratory* system.

The *medical* assistant took the *patient's medical* history.

Physical assessment is an *essential* aspect of *medical* care.

The *Trendelenburg* position is used in cases of shock, in some *abdominal* surgery, and for patients with *low blood* pressure.

Many descriptive adjectives have common endings or suffixes:

Ending	Examples
able	cap*able*, reli*able*
an	Americ*an*
ian	Canad*ian*
al	cervic*al*, occipit*al*, or*al*
ant	const*ant*
eal	periton*eal*
ical	patholog*ical*
ar, ary, ent	muscul*ar*, preval*ent*, pulmon*ary*, transi*ent*, independ*ent*
ese, ful	Chin*ese*, wonder*ful*, care*ful*, cheer*ful*
iac	card*iac*, cel*iac*, man*iac*
ial	influent*ial*, part*ial*
ible, ic, tic	leg*ible*, chron*ic*, epigastr*ic*, thorac*ic*, necro*tic*, hydrochlor*ic*
ior	infer*ior*, anter*ior*, super*ior*
ive, ly	posit*ive*, friend*ly*, comprehens*ive*, manipulat*ive*
ous	delici*ous*, muc*ous*, anxi*ous*
oid, ose	muc*oid*, epiderm*oid*, adip*ose*
ual, y	punct*ual*, tid*y*, chill*y*

A noun may also be used as an adjective. Nouns become adjectives when they are used to describe other nouns.

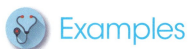 Examples

The *uniform* store went out of business. [The noun *uniform* becomes an adjective because it describes the noun *store*.]

The patient's *blood* pressure is rising slowly.

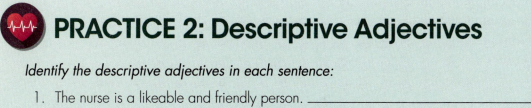 PRACTICE 2: Descriptive Adjectives

Identify the descriptive adjectives in each sentence:

1. The nurse is a likeable and friendly person. _____
2. Clinical examination showed external bleeding. _____
3. Allied health professionals must be responsible employees. _____
4. General procedures should be followed for hospital admission. _____
5. Triangular bandages are used in first aid. _____

PRACTICE 2: Descriptive Adjectives

Placement of Adjectives

The placement of adjectives in a sentence is important to its meaning. To write clearer sentences, place adjectives near the nouns they describe.

- Before the noun: The *doctor's* report was filed correctly. The patient had a *radical* mastectomy.
- After the noun: The report, *exceptional* in detail, provided the necessary information. The doctor, *alert* to physical signs, diagnosed the problem.
- After a linking verb: Just as there is a predicate noun, so, too, there is a predicate adjective. The predicate adjective is found after a linking verb and describes a subject noun or pronoun.
  - He is *apprehensive*. [*Apprehensive* describes the subject pronoun *he* and follows the linking verb *is*.]
  - Shock is *serious*. [*Serious* follows the word *is* and modifies the noun *shock*.]
- At the beginning of a sentence: *Alert* to physical signs, the doctor diagnosed the problem. *Paleness, perspiration,* and *dizziness* are some of the symptoms of this disease.

In a group of adjectives that contains a limiting adjective and one or more descriptive adjectives *that all modify the same noun,* place the limiting adjective first. If there is a noun adjective, it is placed immediately before the noun it modifies.

Limiting Adjective	Descriptive Adjective	Noun Modified	
The	first aid	classes	begin tomorrow.
That	bleeding gunshot	wound	was an accident.

Modifiers and Placement

Modifiers enhance and clarify the meaning of a word. Place the modifier as close as possible to the word it modifies.

A misplaced modifier is out of place and does not modify the word it is meant to modify.

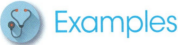
Examples

The doctor had six patients *only* yesterday.

The doctor *only* had six patients yesterday.

The doctor had six patients yesterday *only*.

Consider these sentences with misplaced modifiers:

Misplaced	A medical assistant almost completed all of her procedures.
Revised	A medical assistant completed almost all of her procedures.
Misplaced	The patient in her peritoneal cavity had fluid accumulations.
Revised	The patient had fluid accumulation in her peritoneal cavity.
Misplaced	An ambulance is parked behind the hospital which is out of emergency I.V. fluid.
Revised	An ambulance, which is out of emergency I.V. fluid, is parked behind the hospital.
Misplaced	Give the head injury the anesthetic.
Revised	Give the anesthetic to the patient with the head injury.
Misplaced	Here are some suggestions to improve your illness from the cardiologist.
Revised	Here are some suggestions from the cardiologist to improve your illness.
Misplaced	Demerol was received by the patient of 100 milligrams intramuscularly for the pain.
Revised	The patient received 100 milligrams of Demerol intramuscularly for the pain.

Although many misplaced modifiers result in humor, some could have serious consequences, particularly in legal situations. The court often requests medical records in malpractice cases. Sentences open to various interpretations provide a field day in court that could result in high financial losses.

The way to detect misplaced modifiers is to identify them and rearrange them near the word or words they modify. Read the following examples and note the possibilities for misinterpretation:

 # Examples

Patient is a 40-year-old, white female who came to the emergency room with chest pain at 3:30 a.m. *(Who came to the emergency room, the patient or the pain?)*

The patient called me stating the chest pain was acute prior to the emergency room visit. *(Did the patient call the doctor before the visit, or was the pain acute before the visit?)*

The pain moving toward the neck was located in the right substernal area. *(Was the pain located in the neck or the right substernal area?)*

Now under control with insulin, she has a history of diabetes. *(Is the chest pain or diabetes under control with insulin?)*

Her mother died of myocardial infarction at 45. *(Did the infarction die at 45 or the mother?)*

Here is the paragraph rewritten for clarity:

The patient is a 40-year-old, white female with chest pain who came to the ER at 3:30 a.m. Prior to the ER visit, the patient called me stating the chest pain was acute. The pain was located in the right substernal area and was moving toward the neck. She has a history of diabetes now under control with insulin. The patient's mother died at the age of 45 from myocardial infarction.

PRACTICE 3: Misplaced Modifiers

Revise and simplify these sentences:

1. The computer is in Dr. Kelley's office that doesn't work. _____
2. Buy medicine from the pharmacy with a generic brand. _____
3. The hospital provides comfort for people with central air conditioning. _____
4. The nurse dropped the report I wrote in the wastebasket. _____
5. He was described by a psychotherapist with multiple problems. _____

Degrees of Adjectives to Express Comparison

Degrees of adjectives help describe the quality of a person, place, thing, or idea in comparison to another person, place, thing, or idea. Because qualities vary, adjectives have three different degrees of comparison: the positive, comparative, and superlative.

Positive

The *positive degree* describes nouns *without* making a comparison. The adjective is in its *base* form.

Examples

The hospital has *capable* doctors.   This report is *good*.

Ms. Archer is a *fast* transcriptionist.   Mr. Oberg is *reliable*.

Comparative

Comparative adjectives compare two persons, places, things, or ideas. They are formed in two ways:

1. Add *r* or *er* to the positive or base form of the word. If the word ends in *y*, change the *y* to *i* and add *er*.

Examples

young to young*er*   fat to fat*ter*   tall to tall*er*

happy to *happier*   healthy to health*ier*   smart to smart*er*

The operation was *tougher* than the last one.

This report is *longer* than the pathology report.

Ms. Connolly is *a faster* transcriptionist than the secretary.

2. Add the word *more* or *less* to adjectives of two syllables that do not end in *y* and to adjectives of three or more syllables.

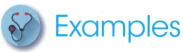 Examples

difficult to *more difficult*   successful to *more successful*

The left ventricle is *more muscular* than the right ventricle.

The patient's medical record is *more reliable* than this letter.

Irregular adjectives are covered later in this chapter under "Other Comparisons."

Superlative

Superlative adjectives are used to compare three or more persons, places, things, or ideas. They usually end in *st* or *est* and are formed in two ways:

1. Add *st* or *est* to the base form of a one-syllable adjective and two-syllable adjectives ending in *y*. If the word ends in *y*, change the *y* to *i* before adding *est*.

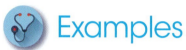 Examples

This lab report is the *longest* one of all the reports.

Your appointment is the *earliest* in the day.

2. Insert the word *most* or *least* before the base form of adjectives of two syllables that do not end in *y* and to adjectives of three or more syllables.

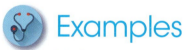 Examples

Mr. Connolly is the *most reliable* medical assistant in the hospital.

The *least important* appointment on the schedule needs to be cancelled.

Dr. Villes is the *most competent* physician in his field.

Some adjectives are irregular. See "Other Comparisons."
The superlative degree may be used for emphasis when there is no obvious comparison.
As a nurse, you are the *greatest*.

PRACTICE 4: Degrees of Adjectives

Indicate the comparative and superlative degrees of these adjectives:

1. weak   _____   _____

2. difficult   _____   _____

3. painful   _____   _____

PRACTICE 4: Degrees of Adjectives

4. dry   _____   _____

5. hearty   _____   _____

Other Comparisons

Some commonly used adjectives are irregular when they form the comparative and superlative degrees:

Positive	Comparative	Superlative
bad	worse	worst
good	better	best
little	less	least
many/much	more	most

Consult a dictionary if you are unsure about the correct word to use.

One of the most common mistakes made in comparisons is using the *double comparison,* or combining *er* with the base word and using *more,* or combining *est* and using *most.*

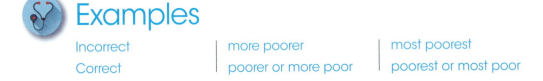 Examples

| Incorrect | more poorer | most poorest |
| Correct | poorer or more poor | poorest or most poor |

Other common mistakes involve the misuse of the words *than* and *as* when making a comparison. *Than* introduces a second person, place, thing, or idea into the comparison.

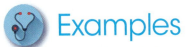 Examples

The right arm is less cyanotic *than* the left arm.

Email is faster *than* sending snail mail.

In expressing both positive and comparative degrees in one sentence, use the word *as* after the positive adjective and the word *than* after the comparative adjective.

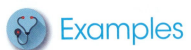 Examples

Your method of filing is *as* well organized, but more complex *than* our method.

The medicine is *as* effective, but less expensive *than* the brand name.

Additionally, do not confuse the word *than* with the word *then*. *Than* is used when comparing modifiers. *Then* means *at that time*.

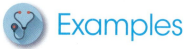

Examples

Your epigastric pain isn't better *than* yesterday's pain?

The incision was made and *then* the retractors were used.

PRACTICE 5: Other Comparisons

Identify the correct comparative degree needed for each sentence:

1. colorful   This hematoma is the _____ of all your bruises.
2. bad   The peptic ulcer is _____ than ever.
3. difficult   The comprehensive exam was _____ than last semester's final.
4. good   Steve is _____ but Dan is _____.
5. competent   The intern is _____, but the specialist is _____.

Troublesome Adjectives

Some adjectives need special attention in their use.

Farther	Refers to distance or a remote point: "Rhode Island is *farther* east than Texas."
Further	Means additional or to a greater extent: *"Further* information is needed before the operation is scheduled."
Later	Refers to the second of two events that occur in chronological order: "The medical assistant reserved a flight *later* in the day."
Latter	Refers to the second of two things presented together: "The doctor could have used OR 1 or OR 2, but decided on the *latter*."
Last	Refers to the final item in a list or series: "The *last* medical payment is due in January."
Latest	Refers to the most recent of something in chronological order: "The Electrocardiograph machine is the *latest* model produced."
Loose	Means free, not tied to something: "Wear *loose* clothing in a wheelchair."
Lose	Means to part with something unintentionally: "The physician did not want to *lose* his stethoscope."

PRACTICE 6: Eponyms

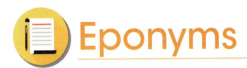

Eponyms

Eponyms are used frequently in medical documentation. An *eponym* is the name of something derived from and identified with a real or mythical person. A medical eponym is the real surname of an individual who is connected with a particular treatment, operation, or instrument. It is very important to spell these eponym adjectives correctly. When in doubt about correct spelling, consult a medical dictionary.

Eponyms are capitalized, but the nouns associated with them are not: Parkinsonism fibers, Bartholin's glands, tetralogy of Fallot, Cheyne-Stokes respirations, Bell's palsy, Babinski reflex, Trendelenburg's position, Epstein-Barr virus, Buck's extension, bundle of His, Fowler's position, DeBakey prosthesis.

PRACTICE 6: Eponyms

Identify the eponyms in each sentence:

1. Patty Grecki in the pediatric ward has a tetralogy of Fallot. _____

2. Was the Babinski reflex in the baby positive? _____

3. Teenagers are sometimes prone to the Epstein-Barr virus. _____

4. Place the patient in a semi-Fowler's position. _____

5. Bell's palsy may sometimes go away within six months. _____

Adjectives Summary

Adjective	Describes a noun or pronoun	
Limiting	Limits the noun or pronoun to a definite or indefinite amount. Answers how many, how much, which one.	a, an, all, any, both, each, every, few, many, more, most, much, no, some, such, that, those, this, these, numbers, possessive nouns, and pronouns.
Interrogative	Asks a question.	which, what.
Proper	Finds its source in a proper noun.	American citizen. Russian immigrant.
Compound	Combines two or more describing words as a single modifier.	state-of-the-art computer (before noun). The computer is state of the art (after noun). over-crowded bus. 5-, 10-, 15-cent stamps.
Predicate	Describes a subject and comes after a linking verb.	The needle is *sharp.* The x-rays are *clear.*
Descriptive	Describes the quality of the person, place, thing, or idea of the noun.	red, large, generous, energetic, partial, beautiful, organized, hungry, poetic, powerful.

Degrees of Comparison Summary

Number of Syllables	Degree			Rule
	Positive (base, describes without making a comparison)	Comparative (compares two or more)	Superlative (compares three or more)	
One syllable	young, new, light	younger, newer, lighter	youngest, newest, lightest	Add *er* or *est* to base.
Two or more syllables	healthy, gentle, expensive, fascinating	healthier, more gentle, more expensive, more fascinating	healthiest, most gentle, most expensive, most fascinating	For words ending in *y*, change *y* to *i* and *er* or *est*. Otherwise, use *more* and *most*.
Irregular adjectives	good	better	best	
	bad	worse	worst	
	little	less	least	
	many	much	most	

Medical Spelling

Become familiar with the spelling of the following words:

abdominal
anterior
antidiuretic
apprehensive
bronchial
calculus, calculi
fetal
frontal
gastrointestinal
hepatic
infection

inguinal
intravenous
lateral
muscular
mucous
myocardial
    infarction
nasogastric
necrotic
pathological
cyanotic

clinical
comprehensive
dorsal
epithelial
excessive
pelvic
peptic ulcer
peritoneal
pleural
proximal
respiratory

retractor
skeletal
streptococcal
superficial
thoracic
tonsillar
uric acid
urinary

Real-World Applications

Medical Reports

Medical reports are very important in the continuity of patient care. They are legal documents. Insurance companies may use them for reimbursements; attorneys may use them in legal suits; providers may use them to affirm a diagnosis. Photographs, digital imaging, scans, and other various integrations of proof and accuracy for the patient's reports are used.

Adjectives play an important role in medical writing, by helping to describe patient conditions and medical procedures and to express degrees of comparison important to medical reports. For example, a patient's chest pain may be moderately severe, or a patient may show *favorable* signs of recovery. Adjectives are also helpful in distinguishing types of reports; for example, radiology reports may often contain terms ending in *-scopy* or *-graphy*. All medical reports contain descriptions of various medical conditions and treatments, so understanding the use of adjectives is essential when writing reports.

Radiology and Imaging Report

A *radiology and imaging report* is a report of what a radiologist interprets from a diagnostic procedure (Figure 4-2). This report is usually filed within four to eight hours of the procedure.

RADIOLOGY REPORT

Patient Name: Marietta Mosley

Hospital No.: 11446

X-ray No.: 98-2801

Admitting Physician: John Youngblood, M.D.

Procedure: Left hip x-ray.

Date: 08/05/20XX

PRIMARY DIAGNOSIS: Fractured left hip.

CLINICAL INFORMATION: Left hip pain. No known allergies.

Orthopedic device is noted transfixing the left femoral neck. I have no old films available for comparison. The left femoral neck region appears anatomically aligned. At the level of an orthopedic screw along the lateral aspect of the femoral neck, approximately at the level of the lesser trochanter, there is a radiolucent band consistent with a fracture of indeterminate age that shows probable nonunion. There is bilateral marginal sclerosis and moderate offset and angulation at this site.

Fairly exuberant callus formation is noted laterally along the femoral shaft.

IMPRESSION: 1. No evidence for significant displacement at the femoral neck.

2. Probable nonunion of fracture transversely through the shaft of the femur at about the level of the lesser trochanter.

_____

Neil Nofsinger, M.D.

NN:xx

D:08/05/20XX

T:08/05/20XX

FIGURE 4-2 Sample Radiology Report

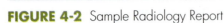

M.A. Novak and P.A. Ireland, *Hillcrest Medical Center Beginning Medical Transcription Course*, 6th ed. Albany, NY: Delmar Thomson Learning, 2005, p. 18.

Examples of such procedures are x-rays, CT (computed tomography) scans, MRIs (magnetic resonance imaging), upper GI series, fluoroscopic studies, nuclear medicine, and ultrasonograms. These medical procedures provide visual images to aid in diagnosis.

Pathology Report

A *pathology report* contains a description of tissue samples removed from the body (Figure 4-3). The removal of a tissue sample for examination is called a *biopsy*. The *pathologist* is the person who studies the tissue samples and generates the pathology report.

PATHOLOGY REPORT

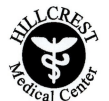

Patient Name: Sumio Yukimura

Hospital No.: 11449

Pathology Report No.: 98-S-942

Admitting Physician: Donna Yates, M.D.

Preoperative Diagnosis: Cholelithiasis.

Postoperative Diagnosis: Cholelithiasis.

Specimen Submitted: Gallbladder and stone.

Date Received: 06/05/20XX

Date Reported: 06/06/20XX

GROSS DESCRIPTION: Specimen received in one container labeled "gallbladder." Specimen consists of a 9-cm gallbladder measuring 2 cm in average diameter. The serosal surface demonstrates diffuse fibrous adhesion. The wall is thickened and hemorrhagic. The mucosa is eroded, and there is a single large stone measuring 2 cm in diameter within the lumen. Representative sections are submitted in one cassette.

GROSS DIAGNOSIS: Gallstone.

KM:xx

D:06/05/20XX

T:06/05/20XX

MICROSCOPIC DIAGNOSIS: Gallbladder, hemorrhagic chronic cholecystitis with cholelithiasis.

_____

Robert Thompson, M.D.

RT:xx

D:06/06/20XX

T:06/06/20XX

FIGURE 4-3 Sample Pathology Report

M.A. Novak and P.A. Ireland, *Hillcrest Medical Center Beginning Medical Transcription Course*, 6th ed. Albany, NY: Delmar Thomson Learning, 2005, p. 20.

The focus of the pathology report is twofold:

1. Macroscopic findings (also called gross description, gross examination). This component describes how the specimen looks to the naked eye. It describes the size, general color, and texture.

2. Microscopic findings (also called microscopic description). This component describes how tissue looks when examined under a microscope.

The report usually ends with a diagnosis of the findings or an impression.

The pathology report is the examination of specific tissues. The pathology report becomes a permanent part of the patient's medical record. A sample pathology report is provided. This report is completed within 24 hours after receiving the laboratory information.

Discharge Summary

The *discharge summary* is a report that is required for all patients who leave the health care facility (Figure 4-4). It is a summary of the patient's condition during his or her stay at the facility. Data in the discharge summary include the following:

- Reason for admittance
- History of present illness
- Social history
- Physical exam and laboratory data
- Events that occurred during the patient's stay
- Follow-up instructions
- Discharge medications

The report concludes with the condition of the patient at the time of discharge and the discharge prognosis. The Joint Commission requires that it be in the patient's chart 48 to 72 hours after discharge from the facility. If the patient expires during the hospital or facility stay, it is then called a "Death Summary."

Operative Report

The *operative report* is a comprehensive description of a surgical procedure performed on a patient (Figure 4-5). The report includes specific details about preoperative, operative, and postoperative experiences such as specimens removed and sent to pathology, diagnosis, type of operation performed, names of surgeons and assistants present, and type of anesthesia, and it may include instruments used, drain packs, closure, sponge count, suture materials and thickness, any unusual circumstances or complications, and estimated blood loss. It is dictated immediately after the operation.

The report may be in narrative form or divided into subheadings, such as "anesthesia," "incision," "findings," "procedures," and "closing." The report details end with the patient going to the recovery room. The operative report must be dictated and filed in medical records as soon as possible after surgery.

DISCHARGE SUMMARY

Patient Name: Joyce Mabry

Hospital No.: 11709

Admitted: 02/18/20XX

Discharged: 02/24/20XX

Consultations: Tom Moore, M.D., Hematology

Procedures: Splenectomy.

Complications: None.

Admitting Diagnosis: Elective splenectomy for idiopathic thrombocytopenic purpura and systemic lupus erythematosus.

HISTORY: The patient is a 21-year-old white woman who had noted excessive bruising since last June. She was diagnosed as having thrombocytopenic purpura. At the same time, the diagnosis of systemic lupus erythematosus was made. The patient continues with the bruising. The patient had been treated with steroids, prednisone 20 mg; however, the platelet count has remained low, less than 20,000. The patient was admitted for elective splenectomy.

LABORATORY DATA ON ADMISSION: Chest x-ray was negative. Electrocardiogram was normal. Sodium 138, potassium 5.2, chloride 104, CO_2 25, glucose 111. Urinalysis negative. Hemoglobin 14.8, hematocrit 43.5, white blood cell count 15,000, platelet count 17,000, PT 11.5, PTT 27.

HOSPITAL COURSE: The patient was taken to the operating room on February 19 where a splenectomy was performed. The patient's postoperative course was uncomplicated with the wound healing well. The platelet count was stable for the first 3 postoperative days. The patient was transfused intraoperatively with 10 units of platelets and postoperatively with 10 additional units of platelets. However, on the fourth postoperative day the platelet count had risen to 77,000, which was a significant increase.

The patient was discharged for follow-up in my office. She will also be seen by Dr. Moore, who will follow her SLE and ITP.

DISCHARGE DIAGNOSIS: Idiopathic thrombocytopenic purpura and systemic lupus erythematosus.

DISCHARGE MEDICATIONS:

1. Prednisone 20 mg q.d.

2. Percocet 1 to 2 p.o. q. 4 h. p.r.n.

3. Multivitamins, 1 in a.m. q.d.

_____

Carmen Garcia, M.D.

CG:xx

D:02/25/20XX

T:02/26/20XX

FIGURE 4-4 Sample Discharge Summary

M.A. Novak and P.A. Ireland, *Hillcrest Medical Center Beginning Medical Transcription Course*, 6th ed. Albany, NY: Delmar Thomson Learning, 2005, pp. 23–24.

OPERATIVE REPORT

Patient Name: Kathy Sullivan

Hospital No.: 11525

Date of Surgery: 06/25/20XX

Admitting Physician: Taylor Withers, M.D.

Surgeons: Sang Lee, M.D., Taylor Withers, M.D.

Preoperative Diagnosis: Urinary incontinence secondary to cystourethrocele.

Postoperative Diagnosis: Urinary incontinence secondary to cystourethrocele.

Operative Procedure: Total abdominal hysterectomy with Marshall-Marchetti correction.

Anesthesia: General endotracheal.

DESCRIPTION: After an abdominal hysterectomy had been performed by Dr. Withers, the peritoneum was closed by him and the procedure was turned over to me.

At this time the supravesical space was entered. The anterior portions of the bladder and urethra were dissected free by blunt and sharp dissection. Bleeders were clamped and electrocoagulated as they were encountered. A wedge of the overlying periosteum was taken and roughened with a bone rasp. The urethra was then attached to the overlying symphysis by placing two No. 1 catgut sutures on each side of the urethra and one in the bladder neck. The urethra and bladder neck pulled up to the overlying symphysis bone very easily with no tension on the sutures. Bleeding was controlled by pulling the bladder neck up to the bone. Penrose drains were placed on each side of the vesical gutter. Blood loss was negligible. The procedure was then turned back over to Dr. Withers, who proceeded with closure.

Sang Lee, M.D.

SL:xx

D:06/25/20XX

T:06/26/20XX

FIGURE 4-5 Sample Operative Report

M.A. Novak and P.A. Ireland, *Hillcrest Medical Center Beginning Medical Transcription Course*, 6th ed. Albany, NY: Delmar Thomson Learning, 2005, p. 19.

Medical Reports Summary

Radiology	A report describing the results of a diagnostic procedure using radio waves or other forms of radiation.
Pathology Report	A report containing a description of tissue samples removed from the body.
Discharge Summary	A report summarizing the patient's condition while at a health care facility.
Operative Report	A report describing a surgical procedure performed on a patient.

Skills Review

Identify any adjectives in these sentences:

1. A streptococcal infection is serious. _____

2. Protein repairs tissues damaged by disease. _____

3. A good trait for a nurse is compassion. _____

4. A pathologist studies diseased tissues. _____

5. Gangrene is obstruction of blood flow resulting in necrotic tissue. _____

Fill in the specific kind of adjective requested:

1. Limiting: _____ staff members work on weekends.

2. Descriptive: Insurance covers only _____ benefits.

3. Interrogative: _____ report do you want faxed?

4. Predicate: The hospital logo was _____.

5. Proper: All _____ citizens must have a social security number.

Write medical adjectives having these suffixes:

1. al _____

2. ian _____

3. ior _____

4. able _____

5. cal _____

6. ic _____

7. ous _____

8. ual _____

9. iac _____

10. ary _____

Circle the correct word within the parentheses in each sentence:

1. Medicine is (most, more) competitive (then, than) it was ten years ago.

2. The hospital is one of the (busy, busier, busiest) facilities in the country.

3. Dr. Swartz is (good, better, best), but Dr. Stevens is (good, better, best).

4. The medical terminology book (further, farther) explains the meaning of words.

5. Over a period of time, (fewer, less) numbers of people applied for the job.

Write true or false next to the following statements:

1. Adjectives answer what kind and how many. _____

2. A noun can be used as an adjective. _____

3. The letters *est* are a sign of the comparative degree. _____

4. The letters *er* are used to describe three or more persons, places, things, or ideas. _____

5. *This, that, these,* and *those* are examples of descriptive adjectives. _____

Grammar Exercise: Underline each error in the paragraph and write its correction above the word.

Based on the evaluation, the patient will be addmitted to the hospital. The patient was placed on a high dose of anti-inflammatory medication. The report concerning the patients abdominal xray were obtained. The patient requiered an intervanous before reaching the hospital. The patients' condition will probably give some pain. This pain can be relieved by over the counter medication. Please call the ofice if there are any questions.

Rewrite these sentences to make them logical:

1. On the second day the knee was better and on the third day it completely disappeared.

   _____

2. The patient left the hospital feeling much better.

   _____

3. The patient has chest pain if she lies on her left side for over a year.

   _____

4. The patient has been depressed ever since she began seeing me ten years ago.

   _____

5. By the time he was admitted, his rapid heart had stopped and he was feeling better.

   _____

Use these words to complete the sentences:

macroscopic findings	pathologist	microscopic findings
pathology report	biopsy	discharge summary
follow-up instructions	paramedic	laboratory

1. The part of the pathology report that describes how tissue looks to the naked eye is _____.

2. The report that documents what happens during hospitalization is _____.

3. The person who examines diseased tissue is a _____.

4. A special report that examines the cause of disease is a _____.

In which medical report may these statements be found?

1. Hospitalized for herniorrhaphy 10 years ago. _____

2. Bleeders were clamped and electrocoagulated as they were encountered. _____

3. Fairly exuberant callus formation is noted laterally along the femoral shaft. _____

4. No evidence for significant displacement at the femoral neck. _____

5. DIAGNOSIS: Gallbladder, hemorrhagic chronic cholecystitis with cholelithiasis. _____

6. I have been asked to see a five-year-old Caucasian male who appears in mild distress due to upper extremity burn after falling into hot coals in his back yard. _____

7. She will be seen by Dr. Kelley, who will follow her systemic lupus. _____

8. Penrose drains were placed on each side of the vesical gutter. _____

Circle the adjectives in the sentences below:

1. The mucosa is eroded, and there is a single, large stone.

2. The patient was admitted for elective splenectomy.

3. Blood loss was negligible.

4. The test showed no evidence of significant displacement at the femoral neck.

5. The patient's postoperative course was uncomplicated.

Circle the correctly spelled word in each line:

1. bronchal   bronchial   bronkial   branchiol
2. cephelic   cefalic   cephalich   cephalic
3. epithelel   epithelial   epathelial   epathelil
4. gastrointestianl   gastrointistinal   gastrointestinal   gastraintistinal
5. mocous   mucos   mucous   nocous
6. pleural   plueral   pleurel   pluerel
7. streptococcal   streptocaccal   stretococcal   streptocacal
8. comprihensive   conprehensive   comprehensive   comprehinsive
9. urinery   uranary   urenery   urinary
10. pathlogical   pathilogical   pathological   patholgical

Comprehensive Review

Underline the adjectives in each sentence. Identify the adjective as limiting, interrogative, proper, compound, predicate, or descriptive:

1. The wall is thickened and hemorrhagic.

2. The patient was taken to the operating room on February 19, where a splenectomy operation was performed.

3. What significant evidence shows displacement at the femoral neck?

4. Functional endoscopic sinus surgery (FESS) was performed by the Mass Eye and Ear specialists.

5. The perioperative nurse should have an empathetic and compassionate ability to care for patients.

Write five sentences involving a medical situation. Use one of each type adjective (interrogative, proper, compound, predicate, or descriptive).

1. _____

2. _____

3. _____

4. _____

5. _____

SECTION 5
Adverbs

Practical Writing Component: Facsimile, Phone Messages, and Minutes of a Meeting

Objectives

After reading this section, the learner should be able to:

- recognize and use adverbs effectively
- distinguish between the use of adjectives and adverbs
- change adjectives into adverbs
- use adverbs to make accurate degrees of comparisons
- avoid the use of double negatives
- place adverbs appropriately
- spell various medical terms
- understand the fax, telephone courtesy and message, and minutes of a meeting

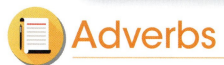 Adverbs

Adverbs are words that modify verbs, adjectives, and other adverbs.

Example modifying verbs:

The patient walked **slowly**. (**Slowly** modifies walked.)

Example modifying adjective:

Ms. Villes is **extremely** respectable. (**Extremely** modifies the adjective respectable.)

Example modifying adverbs:

The white blood cell count rose **exceedingly** rapidly. (Adverb **rapidly** modifies the verb rose and the adverb **exceedingly** modifies the adverb rapidly.)

113

Noun Modifier	Verb Modifier
coronary embolism	*usually* found
axillary crutches	*commonly* used
electrical connection	spoke *eloquently*

Adjectives and adverbs can be distinguished by the different types of questions they answer.

Adjectives Answer:	Adverbs Answer:
Which one	How
What kind	Where
How many how much	When
	How many times
	To what extent

- Adverbs tell *how:* "The details in the chart were described *accurately.*"
- Adverbs tell *where:* "The wound bled *locally.*"
- Adverbs tell *when:* "The operation was performed *yesterday.*"
- Adverbs tell *how many times:* "The nurse cleaned the wound *twice.*"
- Adverbs tell *to what extent:* "Insurance costs increased *dramatically.*"

Examples of Adverbs

actually	early	maybe	seriously
afterward	easily	most	somewhere
again	enough	never	soon
ago	entirely	next	still
almost	especially	now	surely
already	everywhere	obviously	there
always	extremely	occasionally	today
anymore	fast	often	together
anywhere	finally	once	tomorrow
apparently	fortunately	orally	too
carefully	generally	perhaps	up
certainly	hard	quite	very
clinically	here	quietly	well
completely	immediately	rarely	where
constantly	just	regularly	yesterday
downward	later	seldom	yet

If you are confused about whether a word is an adjective or an adverb, determine the part of speech that the word describes. If the word modifies a noun, it is an adjective. If the word modifies a verb, it is an adverb. Note, however, that the same word may be either an adjective or an adverb depending on its use in a sentence:

The nurse gave a *daily* report. [*Daily* is an adjective modifying the noun *report.*]
The nurse administered pills *daily.* [*Daily* is an adverb modifying the verb *administered.*]

 PRACTICE 1: Adverbs

Select the adverb in each sentence and identify the question it answers (how, when, where, how many times, or to what extent):

1. He is extremely frustrated that he cannot use his dentures. _____

2. The cholesterol levels were checked regularly. _____

3. Implants were removed surgically. _____

4. The pain lessened after the patient took the medication. _____

5. The patient took the medication today. _____

 # Adverbs as Modifiers

An adverb is a word that modifies (describes) a verb, verb phrase, adjective, or other adverb. Adverbs that describe verbs are the easiest to identify.

 ## Examples

The patient has recovered *nicely* from the procedure. [*Nicely* modifies the verb *recovered* and answers the question *how.*]

He was casted in the office *yesterday.* [*Yesterday* modifies the verb *casted* and answers the question *when.*]

The medical assistant wrapped the burned area *twice* a day. [*Twice* modifies the verb *wrapped* and answers the question *how many times.*]

Adverbs can also describe adjectives and other adverbs. Examples of adverbs that perform this function are *very, too, rather, fairly, truly, extremely, unusually, exceptionally, somewhat,* and *especially.* Determining whether the adverb modifies an adjective or adverb depends on how the word is used in a sentence.

 ## Examples

The medical team performed an *especially* safe operation. [*Especially* modifies the adjective *safe.*]

The incision healed *fairly* rapidly. [*Fairly* modifies the adverb *rapidly.*]

PRACTICE 2: Adverbs as Modifiers

Identify the adverb(s) in each sentence and state whether the adverb describes a verb, adjective, or other adverb:

1. This elevator services only surgical patients. _____
2. The hospital generally accepts the H&P prepared by the medical office. _____
3. Cranial nerves II-IV appear grossly intact. _____
4. The patient tolerated the procedure well. _____
5. The doctor will probably review the consultation later. _____

Frequency of Adverbs

Specific adverbs exist that describe an amount of time, from full time to no time at all. Some of them are *always, usually, often, sometimes, seldom, rarely,* and *never.*

Examples

I *always* remember. I *sometimes* remember.

I *usually* remember. I *rarely* remember.

I *often* remember. I *never* remember.

The patient *often* reacts to medication. The report is *usually* filed on Mondays. We *always* test the blood for HIV.

Degrees of Comparison

Adverbs, like adjectives, have three degrees of comparison: positive, comparative, and superlative.

Positive

The positive degree shows no comparison. It is the base form of the adverb.

The progress note was written *clearly.*

Comparative

The comparative degree is used to compare two persons or things that perform the same action. Adverbs ending in *-ly* form *comparative degree adverbs* by adding the word *more* or *less* immediately before the adverb. Other adverbs form the comparative by adding *-er* to the base word.

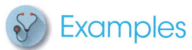

Examples

The progress note was written less clearly than the other one.

James finished the transcription, but Pat did hers faster.

Superlative

The superlative degree is used to compare more than two persons or things that perform the same action. Adverbs ending in *-ly* form *superlative degree adverbs* by adding *most* or *least* immediately before the adverb. Other adverbs are also formed by adding *-est* to the base form.

Examples

The final progress note was written least clearly of all.

The nurse scored the highest in the class.

The hospital admitted patients most cordially.

Irregular Adverbs

Some verbs do not form their comparative and superlative degrees according to the rules stated in the previous paragraphs. They are irregular.

Positive	*little*	Dr. Ramirez cares *little* about covering the emergency room.
Comparative	*less*	Dr. Powers is *less* likely than she to cover the emergency room.
Superlative	*least*	Of all the physicians, Dr. Villmarie is the *least* likely to cover the emergency room.

Other common irregular adverbs are listed below:

Positive	Comparative	Superlative
badly	worse	worst
well	better	best
Much	More	Most

Using Most and More

When using the words *more* or *most,* do not make the mistake of also adding the suffix *-er* or *-est* to adverbs.

Incorrect	Bill worked *more harder* than expected.
Correct	Bill worked *harder* than expected.
Incorrect	Migraines are the most *painfulest* of headaches.
Correct	Migraines are the most *painful* of headaches.

PRACTICE 3: Degrees of Adverbs

Select the correct word in the parentheses:

1. Oral medications are (more, most) acceptable than intramuscular medications.

2. Certified mail is the (good, better, best) way to send documents at the post office.

3. Telecommunication such as a fax machine and computer-to-computer email is the (fast, faster, fastest) method of communication.

4. More medical supplies are (available, more available, most available) on the Internet.

5. The test results are (good, better, best) than they were yesterday.

Changing Adjectives into Adverbs

Medical words can be expressed as adjectives and adverbs.

Examples

The *medical* prognosis for that patient is serious. (Adjective)

The prognosis for that patient is *medically* serious. (Adverb)

1. Simply add -*ly* to the adjective: clinical, clinical*ly*; medical, medical*ly*; physical, physical*ly*; progressive, progressive*ly*; anterior, anterior*ly*; posterior, posterior*ly*; pathological, pathological*ly*.

2. Adjectives that end in *y* preceded by a consonant are made into adverbs by changing the *y* to *i* and adding -*ly*: easy eas*ily*; happy, happ*ily*.

3. Adjectives ending in -*le* are made into adverbs by changing the ending to -*ly*: probable, probab*ly*; acceptable, acceptab*ly*; justifiable, justifiab*ly*.

4. Adjectives ending in *ll* are made into adverbs by adding *y*: full, full*y*; dull, dull*y*.

5. Adjectives ending in *ic* are usually made into adverbs by adding *ally*: historic, historic*ally*; diagnostic, diagnostic*ally*.

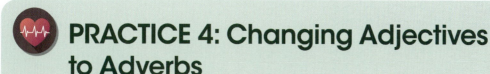

PRACTICE 4: Changing Adjectives to Adverbs

Change the following words into adverbs:

1. safe _____

2. successful _____

3. oral _____

4. continual _____

5. painful _____

Negative Adverbs

A negative, the opposite of affirmative, is a word that expresses a denial or a refusal. A negative contradicts what is said.

> Pedro lives in Boston. [affirmative]

> Pedro does not live in Boston. [negative]

Regular *negative adverbs* are *no, not, never, nowhere, none, hardly, rarely, barely, scarcely,* and *seldom.* Be aware that the word *no* is also a negative *adjective.* Words like *nobody, nowhere, nothing,* and *no one* are negative *pronouns.* The prefixes *dis-, in-, non-,* and *un-* are also indicators of negatives.

Examples

She *never* goes to the doctor. [adverb]

The treatment room has *no* surgical tape. [adjective]

Nobody can tell me the information I want. [pronoun]

Nothing should stand in the way of improving your health. [pronoun]

I did *not* attend the meeting. [adverb]

Unpack the medical supplies that just arrived. [prefix]

The doctor *dis*charged the patient before the weekend. [prefix]

"Not" as a Contraction

The adverb *not* is often joined to verbs to create a new word. The new word is called a contraction. To form a contraction, an apostrophe (') replaces the letter *o* in the word *not* (*n't*). Because the abbreviated form of *not* is implied in the contraction, it is considered a negative word.

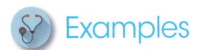

Examples

are not	*aren't*	cannot	*can't*	could not	*couldn't*
might not	*mightn't*	will not	*won't*	would not	*wouldn't*
did not	*didn't*	does not	*doesn't*	do not	*don't*
has not	*hasn't*	have not	*haven't*	had not	*hadn't*
is not	*isn't*	must not	*mustn't*	should not	*shouldn't*
was not	*wasn't*	were not	*weren't*	will not	*won't*

Many people use the contraction *ain't* in their speech. This word is unacceptable in the English language and should not be used. Contractions in general are usually avoided in formal writing.

Double Negatives

Another grammatical error in Standard English is the use of two negatives in a sentence. The rule is two negatives may resolve into a positive. "I do not disagree" could mean "I certainly agree." *Double negatives* should be avoided. Double negatives may decrease the effectiveness of your message and leave an unfavorable or confusing impression.

Incorrect	The policy *didn't* offer *no* deductible.
Correct	The policy offered *no* deductible.
	The policy didn't offer *any* deductible.
Incorrect	The medical assistants *didn't* have *no* money.
Correct	The medical assistants have *no* money.
	The medical assistants *didn't* have *any* money.

Remember double negatives are not effective and are not appropriate in speech or writing.

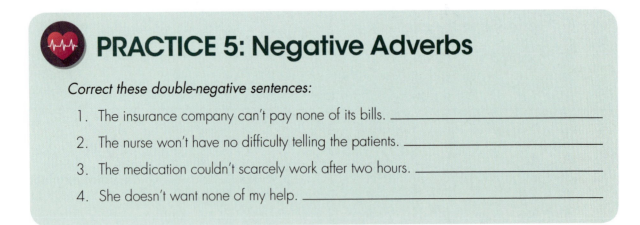

PRACTICE 5: Negative Adverbs

Correct these double-negative sentences:

1. The insurance company can't pay none of its bills. _____

2. The nurse won't have no difficulty telling the patients. _____

3. The medication couldn't scarcely work after two hours. _____

4. She doesn't want none of my help. _____

Placement of Adverbs

If adverbs and adjectives are not placed near the words they describe, they can provide the reader with a good laugh. For example, the sentence "She promised him that she would marry him frequently," should read, "She frequently promised him that she would marry him." Which is the intended meaning: how many times did she promise to marry him, or how many times did she actually marry him?

Adverbs that modify adjectives or adverbs are placed immediately before the words they describe:

Awkward   Luke said that he was going to the office emphatically.

Better   Luke emphatically said that he was going to the office.

Adverbs that modify verbs can be placed in many positions in a sentence:

The doctor listened *intently* to the patient's symptoms.

The doctor listened to the patient's symptoms *intently.*

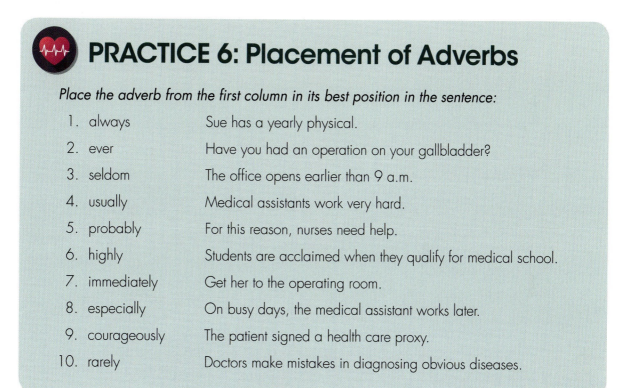

PRACTICE 6: Placement of Adverbs

Place the adverb from the first column in its best position in the sentence:

1. always   Sue has a yearly physical.
2. ever   Have you had an operation on your gallbladder?
3. seldom   The office opens earlier than 9 a.m.
4. usually   Medical assistants work very hard.
5. probably   For this reason, nurses need help.
6. highly   Students are acclaimed when they qualify for medical school.
7. immediately   Get her to the operating room.
8. especially   On busy days, the medical assistant works later.
9. courageously   The patient signed a health care proxy.
10. rarely   Doctors make mistakes in diagnosing obvious diseases.

Troublesome Adverbs

The following words are often confused.

awhile:	The doctor paused *awhile* during the difficult surgery. [adverb]
well:	The patient feels *well*. [adjective]
really:	I was *really* expecting a bonus. [adverb]
surely:	You can *surely* count on me for help when you are ill. [adverb]

a + while:	There was silence in the ER [noun] for *a while*.
good:	The woman had a *good* doctor. [adjective]
real	The patient had a *real* greenstick fracture. [adjective]
sure:	The diagnosis is a *sure* thing. [adjective]

Adverbs Summary

Definition	A word that describes a verb, adjective, or other adverb.	The operation was *successfully* completed.
Question answered	*How? where? when? how many times? to what extent?*	Treatments have to be administered *often*. (how many times)
		The answer may be found *here*. (where)
Placement	Immediately near adjective, anywhere with verb.	What is needed are *extremely* safe guidelines.
Comparative and superlative		
One syllable	Add *er, est*: fast, faster, fastest.	This method is *faster* than the other one.
Two syllables	Add *more, most*: more.	She replied most *impatiently*.
Three syllables	impatiently, most impatient.	
Irregular	*Well, better, best; Badly, worse, worst.*	This is the *worst* I have ever felt.
Avoid double comparatives	Do not use *er* or *est* endings with more and most: more easy *not* more easier; most easy *not* most easiest.	Avoid at all cost.
Avoid double negatives	Do not use two negatives in a sentence (*not, rarely, seldom, hardly, scarcely, barely*).	Avoid at all cost.

Medical Spelling

Become familiar with the spelling of the following words:

abnormally	currently	laterally	primarily
absolutely	developmentally	locally	radically
accurately	dorsally	nutritionally	relatively
analysis	emotionally	occasionally	significantly
apparently	immediately	orally	specifically
axillary	initially	particularly	temporarily
carefully	insufficiently	physically	timely
chronically	intramuscularly	possibly	tomorrow
clinically	intravenously	posteriorly	ventrally
confidentially	involuntarily	potentially	yesterday

Real-World Applications

Fax, Phone Courtesy, Messages, and Minutes of a Meeting

In medical writing, when you describe where and how a procedure was done, how often a treatment was administered to a patient, or to what extent medication is working on a patient's condition, you are using adverbs. Adverbs help to answer questions of how, where, when, and to what extent an action was performed. In the medical setting, sending faxes, taking phone messages, or transcribing the minutes of a meeting may call for this same kind of information and so are good ways to learn the importance of adverbs.

Facsimile

A *facsimile (fax)* is a transmission sent over telephone lines from one fax modem to another fax modem. It is commonly used to send reports and documents in the medical care setting. With the permission of the patient, it is a way to disseminate valuable medical information that is of utmost urgency to medical facilities or a physician. The advantage of transmitting information immediately through the fax lines leads to the enhancement of patient care. HIPAA does require all medical practices to protect health information transmitted over electronic telecommunication lines. Security rules may require encryption for PHI (Protected Health Information). The encryption software security rules are intended to protect personal information transmitted through the Internet. An example of a vitally important fax transmission is the *ECG (electrocardiogram)*. It may be sent to a diagnostician for a reading that could be lifesaving.

A cover sheet should accompany any electronically transmitted message or document. Medical offices have their own cover sheet format that includes all necessary information, as follows:

- the name, phone number, and fax number (or extension, if applicable) of the sender.
- the name, title, department, company, and fax number of the recipient.
- the date the fax is sent and the number of pages.
- any written instructions, messages, or other information.

Figure 5-1 is an example of a fax cover sheet.

Telephone Courtesy and Messages

Telephone etiquette is important in making an impression and setting the stage for patient comfort. Answering the telephone in the medical setting means not only dealing with patients but also with other health care providers. It is important to consider the tone and clarity of one's voice.

Some important points for telephone courtesy:

1. It is always a good policy to use and repeat the patient's name frequently during the telephone call.
2. Write their phone number next to their name.
3. Avoid technical terms.
4. Never put a caller/patient on hold until you know why he or she is calling and receive their permission. It could be an emergency.
5. If returning a call or taking a message, give the caller/patient an idea of when to expect the return call.
6. Never eat or chew gum while on the telephone.

One Morey Place
Anywhere, MA 01102
(555) 555-4727 Phone
(555) 555-444 FAX

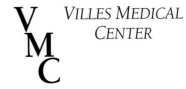

**VILLES MEDICAL
CENTER**

FAX Cover Sheet

To: _Carol LeClaire_   From: _VMC_

FAX: _555-555-4444_   Date: _6-30-20XX_

Phone: _555-4279_   Pages: _7_

(Including cover sheet.)

Comments

The pathology report you requested on Carlos Rodriguez is enclosed.

FIGURE 5-1 Sample Fax Cover Sheet

Most medical offices have an office telephone message pad or appropriate computer screen to maintain a record of all incoming calls or incoming conversations (Figure 5-2). The important thing to remember about phone messages is to deliver them promptly. The efficiency and professionalism of the medical office require that persons receive information in a timely manner.

Information that should be recorded:

1. Date and time of call.
2. Who is the call for?
3. Caller's name, telephone number, and DOB.
4. When can the caller be reached—time and day?
5. Nature of the call? Is it urgent?
6. Message, if any?
7. Call back? Return call? Please call back?
8. Your name please (The one who took the call).

Please repeat the information to the caller to verify that all is correct.
All telephone messages are attached to the patient's medical record.

```
┌─────────────────────────────────────────────────────────────────┐
│  To: Dr. Valerie Christopher                                      │
│                                                                   │
│  Date: 2-18-00                              Time:    9 am         │
│                                                                   │
│                  WHILE YOU WERE OUT                               │
│                  PHONE MESSAGE                                    │
│                                                                   │
│  M      Mark Villes, M.D.                                         │
│                                                                   │
│  Of     Villes Medical Center                                     │
│                                                                   │
│  Phone    555-5551                          Ext 222               │
│                                                                   │
│  _____ Telephoned          _____ Called to see you.     │
│     ✔                                                             │
│  _____ Please call back    _____ Returned your call.    │
│                                                                   │
│  _____ Will call again.    _____ Urgent                 │
│                                                                   │
│  MESSAGE                                                          │
│            Called regarding a metting on March 31 at 5 p.m.       │
│                                                                   │
│                                                                   │
│                                                                   │
│                                                                   │
│                                                                   │
│                                                                   │
│                                                                   │
│                                             Beverly Berc, CMA     │
│                                                                   │
└─────────────────────────────────────────────────────────────────┘
```

FIGURE 5-2 Sample Phone Message

Minutes of a Meeting

Medical personnel may be expected to type the minutes of a meeting. *Minutes* are an official (and sometimes legal) summary record of events and decisions that occur during the meeting. Asking *who, what, where, when,* and *why* about the meeting simplifies the process. All questions need not be answered. These questions are only a tool for getting at the important information. Record only what is done at a meeting and not what is said.

Who	Who attends the meeting? Who is absent? Who is responsible for carrying out tasks? Who chairs the meeting? Who is secretary? Who distributes the minutes? Who reminds people of the next meeting?
What	What happens at the meeting? What decisions are made? What is the meeting about? What is the agenda of this meeting or the next meeting?
Where	Where is the meeting? Where is the next meeting?
When	When is the meeting? When is the follow-up meeting? When does this decision take effect?
Why	Why does the group make the decision? Why are some people absent?

V
M   Villes Medical Center
C   Officer Staff Meeting
          Conference Room
          October 11, 20XX
          2–3 p.m.

Present: Rose William, Office Manager
         Norbert Oberg, RN
         Thomas Buick, Medical Assistant
         Marcia Taft, Secretary

1. The purpose of the meeting was to discuss the distribution of the HIPAA brochures as they pertain to the office staff.

2. Two specific procedures were decided.

3. The brochure will be given to each patient during an office visit.

4. Patients must sign a 506 form verifying receipt of the brochure.

5. These procedures will be evaluated at the December office meeting.

Next Meeting
October 15, 20XX
2–3 p.m.
Conference Room

FIGURE 5-3 Minutes of a Meeting

Like other forms of written communication, a structured model of writing minutes is necessary to ensure a consistent style. Minutes are usually summarized in three components: a heading, a body, and a conclusion (Figure 5-3).

Heading	Name of organization
	Purpose of meeting
	Date, time, and place of meeting
	Chairperson and Secretary
	Names of those present and absent
	Approval of previous meeting's minutes
Body	Paragraph(s) on subject matters regarding decisions, rulings, events, data
Conclusion	Time and place of next meeting
	Agenda
	Chairperson and Secretary

PRACTICE 7: Office Communication

Answer true or false to the following:

1. A cover sheet is not necessary when faxing a message or document electronically. _____

2. If phone messages are recorded, they don't need to be delivered promptly. _____

3. Minutes of a meeting are a summary of events and decisions that occur during the meeting. _____

4. A fax machine is standard equipment in the medical office today. _____

5. Everything that is discussed at a meeting should be included in the minutes of the meeting. _____

 # Fax, Phone Message, and Minutes of a Meeting Summary

Type of Communication	Definition	Format/Structure
Fax	An electronic device that transmits documents, drawings, and photos as exact reproductions	Cover sheet with name, phone number and fax number of sender; name, company, and fax number of recipient; date and number of pages; any message
Phone message	A message from a caller to some one not present to receive the call	Who is the call for, caller's name, phone number, DOB, date, time, purpose of call, when can the caller be reached, message, name of person who took message
Minutes of a meeting	A summary of events and decisions that occur at meetings:	
	Heading	Name of organization
		Purpose of meeting
		Date, time, and place of meeting
		Chairperson and secretary
		Names of those present and absent
		Approval of previous meeting's minutes
	Body	Paragraph(s) on subject matters regarding decisions, rulings, events, and data
	Conclusion	Time and place of next meeting Agenda Chairperson and secretary

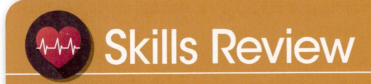

Skills Review

Add to the sentence the type of adverb that is described in the parentheses:

1. The patient ate his meal. (adverb telling how) _____

2. A low-fat diet was ordered. (adverb telling when) _____

3. The patient ambulated to the door and back. (how) _____

4. The pain increased. (how) _____

5. The patient was bleeding. (how) _____

Identify the modifiers and state whether they are adverbs or adjectives:

1. The extensive surgery took hours. _____

2. Xylocaine was used locally. _____

3. The chronic pain was treated with morphine. _____

4. The incision was made laterally. _____

5. The medication was given orally. _____

Give the comparative and superlative forms of these adverbs:

1. fast   _____,   _____

2. badly   _____,   _____

3. lovingly   _____,   _____

4. poor   _____,   _____

5. carefully   _____,   _____

Rewrite these sentences, if necessary:

1. The doctor won't order no laxative.

   _____

2. The patient's temperature hasn't hardly risen all day.

   _____

3. The operation wasn't never cancelled.

   _____

4. Nothing couldn't hardly stop the bleeding.

_____

5. This sphygmomanometer won't never be useful again.

_____

Circle the correct word within the parentheses:

1. The nurse hadn't told (anybody, nobody) about the patient.
2. Occupational Safety and Health Administration, OSHA, standards protect employees who may be (occupational, occupationally) exposed to infectious material.
3. There is exposure to blood or other (potential, potentially) infectious material.
4. The answer to the problem was (probably, probable) easy to solve.
5. Remove all protective clothing (immediate, immediately) upon leaving the work area.

Indicate whether these statements are true or false:

1. The most important procedure in any type of written communication is to follow all steps in the writing process. _____
2. Sending an email is more expensive than using the telephone. _____
3. A cover letter is not necessary when sending a fax. _____
4. Phone messages may be written in longhand. _____
5. Make the email short, complete, and accurate. _____

Circle the correctly spelled word in each line:

1. chronicaly	kronically	chroncally	chronically
2. portnetally	potentiantly	potentially	protentially
3. signifcanntly	signifikantlly	significantly	sigfically
4. intervenously	intrevenously	intervously	intravenously
5. primarely	primarily	premarily	primerily
6. developementally	deveolpmentally	developmentally	defelopmentally
7. imediately	immediately	imediately	immedeately
8. confidentally	confedintialy	confidentilly	confidentially
9. dorsally	dorsilly	dorsaly	dorsully
10. latirally	laterally	latarally	lateraly

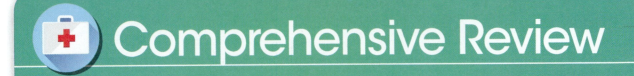

Comprehensive Review

The office medical assistant received a phone call from Dr. Judy Powers at Central Florida Clinics stating that she had a change of plans and cannot attend the conference on this coming Friday morning. She also asked that your employer, Dr. Kelley, call her immediately to reschedule another meeting about the new procedure for wound care.

Use Figure 5-4 to write a phone message to your employer. Include and underline at least three adverbs.

To _____

Date _____ Time _____

WHILE YOU WERE OUT

PHONE MESSAGE

M _____

Of _____

Phone _____

Telephoned _____ Called to see you _____

Please call back _____ Returned your call _____

Will call again _____ Urgent _____

MESSAGE

_____

_____

_____

_____

FIGURE 5-4 Phone Message

Write a different adverb in each circle to modify the verb in Figure 5-5.

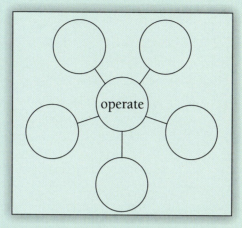

FIGURE 5-5 Adverbs to Modify the Verb

Then write a sentence for each one, using words that apply in a medical situation.

1. _____

2. _____

3. _____

4. _____

5. _____

MODULE 2

Advanced Grammar

SECTION 6
The Sentence
Practical Writing Component: Charting and Documenting

Objectives

After reading this section, the learner should be able to:

- identify the four basic types of sentence structures
- recognize the four classifications of sentences according to their purpose
- identify the factors that contribute to the effectiveness of sentences
- identify independent and dependent clauses
- identify phrases
- identify the factors that cause ineffective sentences
- spell various medical terms
- styles of charting and documenting

 # Introduction

The writing style used in the medical profession is unique. When medical personnel document data, it is usually written without regard to sentence structure. Information is jotted down in abbreviations, words, and symbols. Although abbreviations are used extensively throughout the medical arena, there is movement to limit or keep abbreviations to a minimum. In light of this fact there are certain abbreviations that are prohibited for various reasons. For example, the abbreviation IU (International Units) can be mistaken for IV (intravenous). The Joint Commission website of official "do not use abbreviations" is: http://www.jointcommission.org/facts_about_do_not_use_list/

When abbreviations are translated into formal letters or reports, correct sentence structure is necessary.

Components of the Sentence

Generally, a sentence consists of words that express a complete thought. Sentences contain words, clauses, and phrases. Every sentence contains a subject and a verb. That subject and verb stand independently. It is a thought completed.

Independent and Dependent Clause

A *clause* is a group of words that contains a subject and a verb.

A clause can be *independent* or called the *main clause,* which expresses a complete thought. An *independent* clause can stand alone as a sentence.

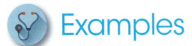 Examples

The nurse gave the medication

Rachelle admitted the patient

A clause can be *dependent.* It can contain a subject and a verb, but does not express a complete thought. A *dependent clause* always begins with a subordinating conjunction or a relative pronoun; it cannot stand alone.

 Examples

because the patient was in pain

before the patient saw the doctor

If you order your prescription today

while she was in the hospital

A complete sentence is made by joining a dependent clause with an independent clause.

 Examples

The nurse gave the medication *because the patient was in pain.*

Rachelle admitted the patient *before the patient saw the doctor.*

If you order your prescription today, you will get a discount.

The patient was too sick to read *while she was in the hospital.*

Examples of subordinating conjunctions are *after, although, as, as if, as long as, as though, because, before, even though, how, if, in order that, provided that, rather than, since, so, so that, though, unless, until, when, whenever, where, whereas, wherever, whether,* and *while.* The relative pronouns are *what, which, that, who, whom,* or *whose.*

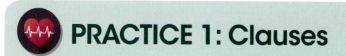

PRACTICE 1: Clauses

Identify the subject of each sentence by asking who? or what? about the verb:

1. The operation was cancelled. _____

2. The patient owns the information in the medical record. _____

3. The physician owns the medical record itself. _____

4. Entries in a medical record are unalterable. _____

5. A breach of confidentiality has legal implications. _____

Identify the dependent clause in these sentences:

1. Medical assistants must use judgment when scheduling appointments that require more evaluation time.

2. The CPT code is assigned for services rendered after a patient has a procedure.

3. While the patient was in the hospital, she developed Pseudomonas.

4. Autoimmune diseases are the cause of many chronic illnesses when a person's self-antigens are damaged.

Types of Dependent Clauses

Noun Clause

The noun clause functions as a noun.

It may be used as a subject, predicate noun, or direct object. Noun clauses are easy to detect because they are introduced by such words as *how, when, where, which, who (whoever), whom (whomever), whose, that, why, what,* or *whether.*

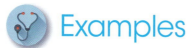

Examples

The doctor didn't know *what* to *say.* [direct object]

Whoever locked the office door must open it. [subject]

What the manager planned was a new hospital wing. [subject]

Adjective Clause

An adjective clause modifies a noun or pronoun. It is usually joined to a main clause by a relative pronoun: *what, which, that, who whose,* or *whom.*

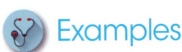 ## Examples

The patient whom the physician diagnosed with cancer left suddenly. [The adjective clause, *whom the physician diagnosed with cancer*, modifies the noun patient.]

A medical assistant *whose name I can't remember* did a great job. [The adjective clause, *whose name I can't remember*, describes the noun *assistant*.]

Adverb Clause

An adverb clause modifies a verb, adjective, or another adverb. They answer the questions *how, when, why, where, how often, to what extent,* and *under what condition* about the verb. They are introduced by subordinating conjunctions.

 ## Examples

Surgeons operate on weekends *if there is an emergency*. [The adverb clause, *if there is an emergency*, modifies the verb *operate*.]

 ## PRACTICE 2: Dependent Clauses

Identify the dependent clauses in each sentence:

1. Aspirin should not be used as an antipyretic with children because it may cause viral problems.
2. Phenylketonuria is a disease in which a hereditary enzyme is absent.
3. The staff was told when the patient arrived.
4. The electrocardiogram provides diagnostic information that the cardiologist needs.
5. When you finish, dispose of the syringes into the proper container.

Phrases

A *phrase* is a group of words without a subject combined with a verb.

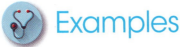 ## Examples

toward the patient's face

in the left kidney

on the operating table

about the curable disease

Prepositional Phrases

A *prepositional phrase* is a group of words that begins with a preposition and ends with a noun or pronoun that is its object. A prepositional phrase can act as an adjective or an adverb.

 # Examples

Adverb phrases:

Fortunately *for the students,* no additional courses were required. [The phrase *for the students* modifies the adverb *fortunately* and answers the question *why*?]

Nurses worked *without a break.* [The phrase *without a break* modifies the verb *worked* and answers the question *how*?]

Adjective phrases:

The procedure *with few side effects* is the best alternative. [*With few side effects* describes the noun *procedure.*]

The pathology report *with tissue results* is due tomorrow. [*With tissue results* describes the noun *report.*]

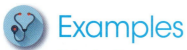 ## PRACTICE 3: Prepositional Phrases

Identify the prepositional phrase in each sentence as adjective or adverb:

1. Unfortunately for the patient, the symptoms indicate glomerulonephritis.
2. The patient went to physical therapy daily.
3. Polyuria is an indication of diabetes mellitus.
4. Urology is the study of the urinary tract.
5. A nephrectomy was performed reluctantly because of kidney failure.

PRACTICE 3: Prepositional Phrases

Participial Phrase

A participle is a verb that is used as an adjective. The phrase consists of the participial (verb) and any modifiers.

 # Examples

The patient, *feeling ill,* took the prescribed medicine. [The participial phrase, *feeling ill,* modifies the noun *patient. Feeling* is the present participle of the verb *feel.*]

The culture *taken from the wound* tested positive for streptococci. [The participial phrase, *taken from the wound,* modifies the noun *culture.*]

PRACTICE 4: Participial Phrase

Identify the participial phrase in each sentence:

1. The sterilized instruments wrapped with tape were removed from the autoclave.

2. The patient's voice, weakened from laryngitis, was barely heard.

3. Physicians experiencing the pressure of the insurance need to take control.

4. Immunizations given throughout childhood are recommended by the Public Health Department.

5. Volunteers, retired from careers, perform valuable services in hospitals.

Gerund Phrase

A *gerund* is a verb form ending in *-ing* that is used in any way that a noun may be used.

 # Examples

Walking is a healthy exercise. [*Walking* is a gerund formed from the verb *walk*, and it is used as the subject of the sentence.]

You can pass this course by *studying*. [The gerund *studying* is used as an object of the preposition *by*.]

Note that both participles and gerunds end in *ing*. The difference is that a participle functions as an *adjective* and a *gerund* functions as a noun.

 # PRACTICE 5: Gerund Phrases

Identify the gerund phrase:

1. Selecting the correct antibiotic is crucial to this infection.

2. Calculating blood gases is an easy process.

3. Analyzing medical information helps to form a diagnosis.

4. Sterilizing instruments under pressurized steam is the most common method of sterilization.

5. Monitoring blood pressure can also be done in a home environment.

Infinitive Phrase

An *infinitive* consists of the word *to* and a verb. It is generally used as a noun, and sometimes as an adjective or adverb.

Examples

Used as a subject	To *operate* would *ease* the pain.
Used as a direct object	The doctor wants *to operate*.
Used as a predicate noun	The decision was *to operate*.
Used as an adjective	The decision *to operate* was made by the.

 ## PRACTICE 6: Infinitive Phrases

Identify the infinitive phrase in each sentence:

1. The nurse practitioner needs to *analyze* the test results.
2. A low fat diet given in small amounts helps to prevent cholecystitis.
3. Leukocytes help to protect the body from infection and tissue damage.
4. To excise the vermiform appendix is called an appendectomy.
5. X-rays are taken to validate any fractures.

 # Sentence Structure

The three sentence structures are simple, compound, and complex.

Simple Sentences

A *simple sentence* has one independent clause and no dependent clause.
   Remember: An independent clause contains a subject and a verb. It expresses a complete thought.

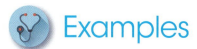 ## Examples

Sutures are surgical stitches.

Patient records are known as charts.

Computerized tomography scans take a series of pictures around the same
   plane.

Compound Sentences

A *compound sentence* contains two or more independent clauses but no dependent clause. The clauses are joined with a coordinating conjunction, a semicolon, or a semicolon and conjunctive adverb. (see notes on punctuation)

Examples

1. Medical asepsis involves procedures to reduce microorganisms, *and* hand washing is the first step in the process.
2. The risks for infection control were raised; the first case of vancomycin-resistant staphylococcus aureus was reported to the Center for Disease Control, CDC.
3. The appointment schedule was booked solid; *therefore,* only emergencies were accepted.

Complex Sentences

A *complex sentence* contains one independent clause and one or more dependent clauses.

Remember: A dependent clause has a subject and a verb but does not express a complete thought. A dependent clause begins with a subordinating conjunction or a relative pronoun.

 # Examples

After the procedure was done, Christopher's major complaint was fatigue.

When preparing for surgical asepsis, the objective is to eliminate all microorganisms.

Whenever a patient complains of chest pain, the first drug given should be aspirin.

Compound-Complex Sentences

A *compound-complex sentence* has two or more independent clauses and one or more dependent clauses. Because they are long, and sometimes difficult to understand, they should be used sparingly.

 # Examples

After being treated with diet restrictions and medications for Crohn's disease, the patient survived, but *he left the hospital with total parenteral nutrition.*

With diabetes being an epidemic in our society, John controls his disease, but *he risks complications with his weight and lack of exercise.*

PRACTICE 7: Sentence Structure

Identify the sentences as either simple, compound, or complex.

1. Many supplies in the doctor's office are disposable, and many are made of surgical steel for autoclaving. _____

2. When one is preparing for surgical asepsis, the objective is to eliminate all microorganisms. _____

3. Autoclaving is the most common method of sterilizing. _____

4. Keep charts neat. _____

5. Sterile solutions are often required during surgical procedures. _____

Classifications of Sentences

Sentences are classified in four ways according to what they do: declarative, imperative, interrogative, and exclamatory.

Declarative Sentences

Most sentences are declarative because they make known (*declare*) some type of information or statement. A *declarative sentence* ends with a period (.).

 ## Examples

The medical assistant is responsible for filing.

The diagnosis is influenza.

A differential diagnosis is given when there are other possible diagnoses.

Pulse oximetry revealed an oxygen saturation of 83%.

The record will be organized according to the needs of the physicians.

Imperative Sentences

Imperative sentences give a command or make a request. In an imperative sentence, the word *you* is understood as the subject, even though it is not written. Imperative sentences end with a period (.).

 ## Examples

Transcribe the History and Physical in full block form.

Make the margins one inch on either side of the report.

Photocopy the correspondence and file it.

Fax this consultation letter to Dr. Villes.

Make the follow-up appointment in one week.

Interrogative Sentences

Interrogative sentences ask direct questions and end with a question mark (?).

 ## Examples

Did you include the name of the patient and the reason for the appointment?

What is the etiology of that disease?

Do you know the difference between exocrine and endocrine?

What is the Joint Commission?

How are charting errors changed or corrected?

Exclamatory Sentences

Exclamatory sentences express strong emotions and end with an exclamation point (!).

 ## Examples

The patient is in cardiac arrest!

Call 911!

Prepare the operating room now!

Look at the size of that tumor!

 ## PRACTICE 8: Classifications of Sentences

State whether the following sentences are declarative, imperative, interrogative, or exclamatory:

1. Does your family have a history of cancer? _____

2. Epinephrine now! _____

3. Leave a message at the tone. _____

4. Eliminate the allergens to reduce the asthma attacks. _____

5. Anxiety is a normal response to surgery. _____

 # Effective Sentences

Writing for medical professionals is very different from other professions. A person's reason for writing greatly influences the tone or manner in which words are expressed. A novelist uses multiple words to create settings, establish moods, and express emotions. A historian concentrates on exact times, cultures, and the cause and effect of events. A poet uses metaphors, rhythm, and rhyme. Medical writers use abbreviations, codes, and phrases unique to their situations. Note the difference in style between a novelist and a medical professional (Table 6.1).

TABLE 6-1   Style Between a Novelist and a Medical Professional

Novelist	Medical Professional
How glad she was to see her children! She wept for pleasure when she felt their little arms clasping her; their hard, ruddy cheeks pressing against her own glowing cheeks. She looked into their faces with hungry eyes that could not be satisfied with looking. [Kate Chopin, *The Awakening*]	Patient experiences no motion in the back. Range of motion of the hips is within normal limits and painless. There is only a +1 dorsalis pedis on the right; otherwise, there are no peripheral pulses present. There is marked coldness of both feet. [Diehl and Fordney *Medical Typing and Transcribing*]

Many elements contribute to the effectiveness of good sentence structure. Four of these elements are covered in this chapter: parallel structure, conciseness, word choices, and positive statements.

Parallel Structure

Parallel sentence structure requires that words, phrases, and clauses be expressed in the same grammatical construction. The elements or units of a sentence (words, phrases, and clauses) joined by a conjunction should be expressed in the same form. The sentence reads smoothly when the ideas are expressed in this cohesive way.

 ## Examples

a noun with a noun	*doctors* and *nurses*
an adjective with an adjective	*red* and *green* lights
an infinitive with an infinitive	*to* speak and *to* listen
a gerund with a gerund	*climbing* and *reaching*

 ## Examples

Nonparallel	Dr. Spencer is *trustworthy* and *a gynecologist*. [*Trustworthy* is an adjective and *gynecologist* is a noun.]
Parallel	Dr. Spencer is a *surgeon* and a *gynecologist*. [two nouns]
Parallel	Dr. Spencer is *trustworthy* and *honest*. [two adjectives]
Nonparallel	The medical assistant's tasks are *transcribing* and *to file*. [*Transcribing* is a gerund and *to file* is an infinitive.]
Parallel	A medical assistant's tasks are *transcribing* and *filing*. [two gerunds]
Parallel	A medical assistant's tasks are *to transcribe* and *to file*. [two infinitives]

 ## PRACTICE 9: Parallel Structure

Identify these sentences as parallel or nonparallel:

1. The patient underwent minor surgery, an X-ray, and blood test. _____

2. The patient education was interesting and of knowledge. _____

3. The doctor proofread the History and Physical quickly and thoroughly. _____

4. I want an appointment for next week, rather than putting it off until next month. _____

5. Ann purchased a computer, a color printer, and she also bought a modem.

   _____

Conciseness

Conciseness is the hallmark of medical documentation. *Conciseness* is expressing a lot of information in a few words. More words are not necessarily better. Sentences should not be cluttered with unnecessary words.

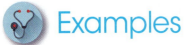 Examples

Wordy	The black and blue mark is on the right lower leg.
Concise	The hematoma is on the right lower leg.
Wordy	If you think you want more information, don't hesitate to call.
Concise	Call me for more information.
Wordy	The purpose of this letter is to acknowledge the receipt of your medical payment.
Concise	Thank you for your remittance.
Wordy	We received your check for the full amount.
Concise	We received the balance in full.
Wordy	The patient has difficulty breathing.
Concise	The patient has dyspnea.
Wordy	To the best of my knowledge, we did all we could do for the patient.
Concise	We did all we could for the patient.

> A sentence should contain no unnecessary words, a paragraph, no unnecessary sentences, for the same reason that a drawing should have no unnecessary line and a machine no unnecessary part.
>
> William Strunk, Jr.

Wordy expressions can be replaced by concise words (Table 6.2).

TABLE 6-2 Wordy Expressions	
Wordy Expressions	**More Concise**
as a result	therefore
at this time, at this point in time	now, currently
bring to a conclusion	conclude, end
cognizant of the fact	know
due to the fact that	because
during the month of	during
each and every	each

Wordy Expressions	More Concise
enclosed please find	I am enclosing
lend credence to the report	support the report
many eccentricities	many behaviors
peruse the document	read the document
I would appreciate it if	please
in regard to	regarding, concerning
in some cases	sometimes
in reference to the subject matter	regarding
in the near future	soon
it has come to our attention	we learned
it is incumbent on you	it is your duty
of primary importance	significant
please be advised that	know
regarding the matter of	regarding

To be concise also means to reduce the length of sentences. Writing shorter sentences means using fewer words. Ten or fifteen words per sentence is about average. Be careful of sentences that run longer than two typed lines. Shorten lengthy sentences by adding periods and making two or more sentences out of one (see the following examples).

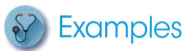 Examples

Lengthy Sentence	The gallbladder was edematous and somewhat thick-walled, with a stone lodged in the cystic duct of the gallbladder, measuring about 1.0 cm in diameter, but there were no filling defects and there was good emptying of the contrast medium into the duodenum.
Revision	The gallbladder was edematous and somewhat thick-walled. It contained a 1.0-cm stone lodged in the cystic duct of the gallbladder, which had no filling defects.

Eliminate unnecessary words. Write to express, not impress.

On the other hand, too many short sentences could be boring:

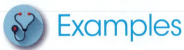

Examples

Short Sentences	Heather Adams is an 83-year-old woman. She also looks young for her age. She has a history of heart problems. She refused medication. It makes her dizzy. There are also occasional accidents from incontinence. Also diarrhea. X-rays were ordered.
Varied Sentences	Heather Adams is an 83-year-old woman with a history of heart problems. She refuses medication because it makes her dizzy. The patient experiences incontinence and diarrhea. X-rays were ordered.

Another way to be concise is to change a dependent clause into either a phrase, an appositive, or a single word.

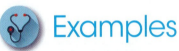

Examples

Phrase (a group of words without a subject or verb predicate)

Working medical staff [gerund phrase]

After the operation [prepositional phrase]

To get an early start [infinitive phrase]

Troubled by headaches [participial phrase]

Appositive (a word or group of words that renames)

Louis, who is the physical therapist = Louis, the physical therapist

Single Word

That had been canceled = canceled

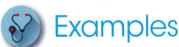

Examples

Clause	The biopsy *that came to the pathology laboratory* was not scheduled for today.
Phrase	The biopsy *from the pathology lab* was not scheduled for today.
Clause	*After you graduate,* you are eligible for the certification exam.
Phrase	*After graduation,* you are eligible for the certification exam.
Clause	Her two nurses, *one of whom is Joan and the other Bill,* took care of her.
Appositive	Her two nurses, *Joan and Bill,* took care of her.
Clause	Allow the patient *who is angry* to express his feelings.
Single Word	Allow the *angry* patient to express his feelings.

PRACTICE 10: Conciseness

Make these sentences more concise:

1. You are eligible for Medicare because of the fact of your age. _____

2. The pharmacy makes deliveries of customers' medications for a charge that amounts to $7.00 per delivery. _____

3. The group moves to negotiate acceptance of the physician's plan. _____

4. During the month of April, my health premiums increased by the amount of 5%. _____

5. Enclosed please find a check in the amount of $100. _____

Keep the meaning of these sentences, but make them more concise:

1. In progress notes, some doctors write in longhand that is hard to read. _____

2. The patient had herpes zoster at a young age and recovered nicely. _____

3. The patient is alert, holding the right section of his arm at times during the exam. _____

4. Prompt diagnosis and treatment comes from early recognition of signs and symptoms. _____

5. When original materials are used in a report, credit must be given to the author in a footnote. _____

Diction

Diction refers to the writer's choice of words and how those words are used in writing. Diction makes the difference between a clear style and a weak, vague style. The intended audience usually determines the type of diction. Among the types that have no place in medical documentation are unfamiliar words, slang, colloquialisms, and vagueness.

Some writers feel that using long or unfamiliar words makes a good impression. Although these words have their merit, medical documentation is not the place to impress.

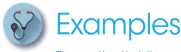 ## Examples

The patient's *idiosyncrasies* irritated her condition.

The patient's *behavior* irritated her condition.

Peruse the medical report before you make any comment.

Read the medical report before you make any comment.

Slang is a new or old expression that contains colorful words and expressions that take on new meaning. Phrases like *don't bug me, it's cool, in the swim,* and *off the wall,* are examples of slang. Colloquialisms are informal words and phrases used in everyday conversation: *globs, lots and lots, all revved up,* and *been there–done that.*

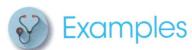 # Examples

The patient is off the wall.

Medical research is not my thing.

The new medical equipment is real cool.

Another trap to avoid in writing effective sentences is the use of vague words or phrases. Vagueness is expressing oneself unclearly. Like slang and colloquialisms, vague words have no place in medical documentation. Recording that a patient received medication without the name or dosage of the drug opens the door to all kinds of problems. Can you imagine the consequences if a medical assistant failed to document that a patient's *right* hand was the source of pain? Be specific with the facts. Assume nothing in medical reporting. Use specific words over vague words or wordy expressions.

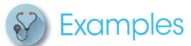 # Examples

Vague	The patient wasn't feeling well.
Specific	The patient complained of abdominal pain. His skin was cool, pale, and moist.
Vague	The head nurse supervised the project.
Specific	Ellen Barker, the head nurse, supervised the Ethics Project.
Vague	Call me some time during the day.
Specific	Call me between 1:00 and 2:00 P.M. on Wednesday.

> The difference between the right word and the nearly right word is the same as that between lightning and the lightning bug.
>
> Mark Twain

 # PRACTICE 11: Diction

Underline the sentence in each pair that provides specific information:

1. A. Come to the office tomorrow.

   B. Make the appointment on Wednesday at 3:15 P.M.

2. A. The physician informed the Board of Directors about the financial situation.

   B. Last night, the patient had lots and lots of pain and discomfort.

3. A. You and I think along the same lines.

   B. The moral issue about confidentiality was discussed at the meeting.

4. A. Credit was given to Dr. Sullivan for his consultation report.

   B. Although many suggestions were good, some were very far out.

5. A. The patient could care less about what medication to take.

   B. I appreciate the effort you put into fund raising.

Positive Statements

To write more effective sentences, use positive statements instead of negative ones. Write what can be done rather than what cannot be done. A positive tone creates an environment of efficiency, acceptance, and professionalism. Notice how these negative sentences were changed to positive sentences:

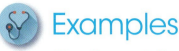 Examples

Negative	Your medication isn't due until 3 P.M.
Positive	Your medication is due at 3 P.M.
Negative	Why didn't you clean the wound before applying bacitracin?
Positive	Clean the wound well before applying the bacitracin.
Negative	The medication isn't in stock right now.
Positive	We expect to receive the medication tomorrow.
Negative	You did not sign the release form.
Positive	Please sign the release form.

Negative sentences, like those used in the previous examples, contain some form of the word *not*. Other negative words are *nor, never,* and *no*. Some sentences may also convey a negative tone even without using a specifically negative word.

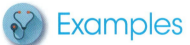 Examples

Negative	Doctors are like God.
Positive	Doctors are human like everyone else.
Negative	Get it right the first time.
Positive	I'll take my time and do it well.
Negative	What if I lose my job?
Positive	If I lose my job, I'll find a better one.

 PRACTICE 12: Positive Sentences

Change these negative sentences to positive ones:

1. Most people never change. _____

2. My supervisor refused to give me a raise. _____

3. The doctor's office isn't open after 5 P.M. _____

4. You won't be satisfied with the quality of care in that hospital. _____

5. Don't think twice about calling the doctor. _____

Ineffective Sentences

A poorly constructed sentence is one that disrupts the smooth flow of a clear message. Three common constructions that cause ineffective sentences are fragmented sentences, comma splices, and run-on sentences.

The Fragmented Sentence

Sentences that do not express a complete thought are called *fragmented sentences* because some necessary information is omitted. *Fragmented sentences* occur when a phrase or a dependent clause is erroneously punctuated as though it were a complete sentence.

 ## Examples

Because of medical staff absenteeism.

If you want to stay healthy.

Medical x-rays that indicate.

Medications in the locked closet.

The preceding examples are dependent clauses. Additional information must be added to make complete sentences. Notice that fragmented sentences may contain a subject and verb; however, they depend on other clauses to give meaning to the sentence.

 ## Examples

Because of medical staff absenteeism, everything was behind schedule.

If you want to stay healthy, drink more water and exercise daily.

Medical x-rays that indicate an abnormality in the neck require further review.

Medications in the locked closet need to be distributed.

Edit, revise, and proofread each sentence until it is clear and complete.

 ## PRACTICE 13: Incomplete Sentences

State whether these sentences are complete or fragmented:

1. Recording each patient's medication. _____

2. Common charting terminology. _____

3. Use plastic gloves for aseptic reasons. _____

4. Decontaminate work surfaces. _____

The Comma Splice

A *comma splice* occurs when two or more independent clauses are incorrectly connected by a comma.

 # Examples

First we cleaned the incision, then we did the dry sterile dressing.

Migraines occur when the vessels are not filled with blood, the scalp feels the pain.

The patient can waive confidentiality, confidentiality can also be overruled through a court order or subpoena.

The Run-On Sentence

A *run-on sentence* occurs when two or more independent clauses are joined together without punctuation.

Examples

First we cleaned the incision then we did the dry sterile dressing.

Migraines occur when the vessels are not filled with blood the scalp feels the pain.

The patient can waive confidentiality confidentiality can also be overruled through a court order or subpoena.

The run-on sentence and the comma splice can be corrected in the following ways:

1. Connect the independent clauses by a comma and a coordinating conjunction.

    First we cleaned the incision, and then we did the dry sterile dressing.

    Migraines occur when the vessels are not filled with blood, and the scalp feels the pain.

    The patient can waive confidentiality, but confidentiality can also be overruled through a court order or subpoena.

2. The independent clauses can be put into two separate sentences.

    We cleaned the incision. Then we did the dry sterile dressing.

    Migraines occur when the vessels are not filled with blood. The scalp feels the pain.

    The patient can waive confidentiality. Confidentiality can also be overruled through a court order or subpoena.

3. A semicolon can connect the closely related clauses. Sometimes a conjunctive adverb is used.

    First we cleaned the incision; then we did the dry sterile dressing.

    Migraines occur when the vessels are not filled with blood; consequently, the scalp feels the pain.

    The patient can waive confidentiality; however, confidentiality can also be overruled through a court order or subpoena.

4. Make one of the independent clauses into a dependent clause.

    After we cleaned the incision, we did the dry sterile dressing.

    Migraines occur when the vessels are not filled with blood, while the scalp feels the pain.

    Although the patient can waive confidentiality, confidentiality can also be overruled through a court order or subpoena.

Poor punctuation is the only cause of run-on sentences. By not using a period, semicolon, or conjunction, one sentence is permitted to run into another. Carelessness rather than a lack of understanding more likely causes this type of error.

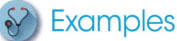 # Examples

Run-on	I took her vital signs I marked the results on the patient's chart. [No punctuation mark or coordinating conjunction used between the two complete sentences.]
Correct	I took her vital signs. I marked the results on the patient's chart. [A period separates the two sentences.]
Correct	After I took her vital signs, I marked the results on the patient's chart. [Revised to make a single sentence with a dependent and independent clause.]
Run-on	I took her vital signs, I marked the results on the patient's chart. [A comma is used in place of a period.]
Correct	I took her vital signs, and I marked the results on the patient's chart. [Added a coordinating conjunction.]

PRACTICE 14: Comma Splice and Run-on Sentences

Identify the following sentences as true or false:

1. A run on sentence occurs when independent clauses are joined without punctuation. _____

2. The predicate of a sentence tells who or what about the verb. _____

3. A sentence forms a dependent clause. _____

4. A sentence fault disrupts the flow of ideas. _____

5. Independent clauses can form two sentences. _____

 # Sentence Summary

Clauses Summary

| Clause: | A group of words containing a subject and verb. Independent clauses contain a subject and a verb, express a complete thought, and can exist alone as a sentence. Dependent clauses contain a subject and a verb but do not express a complete thought and cannot exist alone in a sentence. |
| | Dependent clauses are introduced by subordinating conjunctions and relative pronouns: |

Subordinating Conjunctions	Relative Pronouns
after, although, as, as if, as long as, as though, because, before, even though, how, if, in order that, provided that, rather than, since, so, so that, that, though, unless, until, when, whenever, where, wherever, whereas, whether, while	which, that, who, whom, whose, what

Function	Identifier	Example
Noun used as a subject, predicate noun, or direct object.	Introduced by how, when, where, which, who, whoever, whom, whomever, whose, that, why, what, whether.	The wheelchair is *what I ordered.* I know *how you are feeling.*
Adjective used to tell *which one* or *what kind.*	Often introduced by a relative pronoun: *which, that, who, whom, whose, what.*	That was the house *where Dr. Brown lived.* Supplies, *which were ordered in May,* have not arrived yet.
Adverb used to tell about a verb, adjective, or another adverb.	Introduced by *also, because, beside, for example, however, if, in addition to, instead, meanwhile, then, therefore.*	She practices *because she wants to be a better pianist.* *If you discover a fire,* ring the alarm immediately.

Phrases Summary

Phrase: A group of words without a subject or predicate, which functions as a noun, adjective, or adverb in a sentence.

	Composition	Function	Example
Prepositional phrase	Begins with a preposition, plus nouns or pronouns and any modifiers	Group of words that acts like a single modifier.	. . . valve *in the heart* . . . . . . parking lot *behind the hospital* . . . . . . time *at your earliest convenience* . . .
Used as an adjective	Begins with a preposition, plus nouns or pronouns and any modifiers	Modifies a noun or pronoun. Answers *which one? what kind? how many?*	. . . the blood *in the heart* . . . . . . medicines *to cure infections* . . .
Used as an adverb	Begins with a preposition, plus nouns or pronouns and any modifiers.	Modifies a verb, adjective, or other adverb. Answers *how? what? where? when? why? to what extent?*	The blood flowed *through the aorta.* The doctor operated on *weekends.* Nurses worked *around the clock.*

Verbal Phrase: A group of words including a verbal and its subject, object, complement, or modifiers that function as a noun, adjective, or adverb.

	Composition	Function	Example
Participial	Begins with a verb ending in *ing* (present participle) or in *t, d, ed, en* (past participle).	Adjective	Nurses *dedicated to patient care are* unsung heroes. The report *containing the patient's history* was sent to another hospital.
Gerund	Begins with an *ing* verb and includes any modifiers.	Noun	*Eating healthy food* is an excellent habit. An excellent habit is *eating healthy food.*
Infinitive	Begins with *to*, plus present form of a verb and any modifiers.	Noun, predicate noun, adjective, or adverb	*To question* is a sign of intelligence. The doctor asked *to see the file.*

Sentence	Subject (Simple or Compound)	Complete Subject	Simple Predicate (Verb)	Complete Predicate
My sister, Ethel, is a technician.	Ethel (simple subject)	My sister, Ethel	is	is a technician.
Dental care is free to children.	care (simple subject)	Dental care	is	is free to children.
The hurricane and wind destroyed many houses and trees.	hurricane and wind (compound subject)	The hurricane and wind	destroyed	destroyed many houses and trees.

Sentence Structure

Simple Sentence	Contains one independent clause.	The disease was contagious.
Compound Sentence	Contains two or more independent clauses.	The disease was contagious, but precautions were taken.
Complex Sentence	Contains one independent clause and one dependent clause.	Careful handwashing reduces the spread of contagious disease when done properly.

Classifications of Sentences

Declarative	Makes a statement, is used more than any other type, and ends in a period: "This doctor seldom asks for a copayment."
Imperative	Gives a command, makes a request, and ends in a period. The subject *you* is understood: "Give the patient medicine." "Don't forget your appointment."
Interrogative	Asks a question and ends with a question mark: "What is my temperature?" "When are you flying to France?"
Exclamatory	Expresses strong feelings and ends with an exclamation point: "Get to the ER quickly!"

Characteristics of Effective Sentences

Parallel structure	Two or more sentence elements of equal rank expressed similarly: "Water skiing is as challenging as to dive" [not parallel]. "Water skiing is as challenging as diving" [parallel].
Conciseness	Avoiding wordiness and sentences that are too long: "We were sitting in seats that were close to the stage" [wordy]. "We were sitting close to the stage" [concise].
Appropriate diction	Clear expression through the choice of words and how they are used in a sentence: "The meeting is in the afternoon" [vague]. "The team meeting is at 3:30 p.m." [precise].
Positive statements	Affirmative expression: "I can't perform that procedure" [negative]. "I'll refer you to a physician who does that procedure" [positive].

Ineffective Sentences	
Fragment	Does not express a complete thought and occurs when a phrase is considered as a sentence: "involuntary shaking," "under medical care," "who are known to have hemophilia."
Run-on	Omits punctuation between two sentences: "Chart notes are formal or informal physicians take them when they see a patient." "The abdomen is flat without scars bowel sounds are normative." "Make an entry in the chart do the entry correctly."
Comma Splice	Incorrectly uses a comma to connect two or more independent clauses: "The goal of organizing documents is to provide easy access to patient information, information is needed by many different health professionals."

Medical Spelling

Become familiar with the spelling of the following words:

assessment	endogenous	insomnia	pediculosis
cachexia	endoscopy	integrity	perceptual
carcinogens	enteric	interferon	pericarditis
chemotherapeutic	episodic	interstitial	rehabilitation
cytology	evisceration	intoxication	stenosis
dehiscence	exacerbation	manifestation	syndrome
dementia	fissure	mediastinum	tolerance
diabetes	fluoroscopy	narcolepsy	ultrasound
diffusion	immunoglobulins	neurophysiologic	vitiligo
dysplasia	incontinence	oxygenation	visceral
emesis	influenza	pathophysiology	

Real-World Applications

Progress Notes, Charting, and Documenting

Chart notes, nurse's notes, and progress notes are a description detailing the encounter specifics of a connection with a patient. They are what we see, feel, hear, measure, and count. They are never what we assume. They are permanent. They are legal. They are part of the medical record. They are in chronological order. It helps the medical team understand what was done, what needs to be done, and what is planned for patient care. The documentation also provides proof that one has provided care to the patient. There is an adage in nursing that states, "If it was not charted, it was not done." Documentation is also used for billing and reimbursement of services.

There are many types of charting. The method for your facility is the method that should be followed. Now that the electronic records are used more frequently some doctors and nurses are rethinking the order of information disclosed and the use of SOAP notes. There has been a migration from paper records to hybrids of the electronic medical record. Maintaining and functioning electronic medical records are different in every office situation.

Some important points:

1. Never document care before it is given.
2. Never leave blank spaces between notes.
3. Do not criticize care that was given.
4. Do not chart anything you did not witness/or chart for someone else.

The medical assistant can write only what is observed or what is seen. What is observed is called "Objective." What is seen is called "Subjective." These are often referred to as "S" and "O."

Using phrases and clauses for:

1. the chief complaint—what is the patient complaining of?
2. the location of the problem—where is the pain?
3. quality—type of pain, is it sharp, dull?
4. the severity of the pain—on a scale of 1 to 10, how severe is the pain?
5. duration—how long does it last?
6. timing—how often does the pain occur?
7. context—how, when, where did it happen?
8. modifying factors—is it better elevated or with ice or heat applied?
9. other signs or symptoms?

Traditional Charting

Notes are phrases, clauses, and sentences without any specific structure. For example, "the patient is comfortable, visitors today."

This type of information is often placed in the source-oriented medical record (SOMR). It is a simple system and requires the least amount of work and organization.

SOAP

Lawrence Weed, M.D., instituted the *problem-oriented medical record (POMR)* method in 1969, at Case Western Reserve in Cleveland. The POMR organizes the patient's record in a comprehensive manner by charting the patient's problems in order of importance and how those problems are addressed. Some institutions still use this format. Others have incorporated part of the format to fit their own charting and documenting needs. The POMR has four parts:

1. *Data base.* The data consists of information from various sources that identifies the problem and is the basis for evaluating the patient's health.
2. *Problem list.* This is a chronological list of the patient's problems and reasons for seeing the doctor.
3. *Initial plan.* A treatment plan is developed to address each problem the patient has.
4. *Progress notes.* The written notes are called *SOAP* (Subjective-Objective-Assessment-Plan) notes (Figure 6-1). In this format, progress notes are dated, headed, and numbered for specific problems.

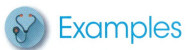 Examples

SOAP notes consist of:

S Subjective—record what the patient says, such as nausea, description of symptoms and feelings.
I have a pain in my leg.
The patient complained of pain in the lower back.
Patient complained of migraine headache.

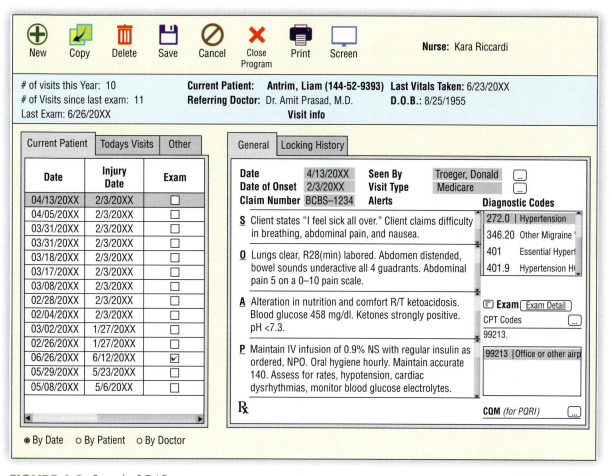

FIGURE 6-1 Sample SOAP note

O Objective—record what the doctor, nurse, or medical assistant observes.
results from tests and physical exam.
weeping, inflammation, vital signs.

A Identify a diagnosis—An assessment by the physician/provider, with impressions.
arthritis of the leg
Diagnosis: *emphysema*
Patient has chronic bronchiolitis.

P A treatment plan or medical intervention for medical problems—includes medications, consults, surgery, and patient education.
Take aspirin every 4 hours for pain.
Patient to physical therapy three times a week.

If, for instance, a patient comes to the emergency room and is complaining of being hot, and is perspiring and flushed, the medical assistant may enter the following information. The entry might read like this:

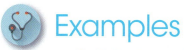 Examples

S—Patient complains of temperature and diaphoresis.
O—Vital signs taken: T-102, P-80, R-24, B.P 150/80, diaphoretic.
A—(Assessment information: to be completed by physician/provider.)
P—(Treatment plan/medical intervention recommended: to be completed by physician/provider.)

SOAPE

SOAP notes were later modified to include evaluation:

E	An evaluation stating how the patient responded to the illness and reacted to the treatment, medications, and medical care.

SOAPIE

Another system added intervention and its evaluation:

I	Implementation or how the actions were carried out: an approach to a particular problem.
E	The evaluation or the report of the actual patient outcome or the response of subsequent treatment.

SOAPIER

Other components to the SOAP system of charting include intervention, evaluation, and revision.

I	Implementation or the approach to a particular problem.
E	Evaluation looks at the patient's response to the treatment intervention.
R	Revision identifies changes that are prompted by the evaluation.

PIE

PIE (Problem–Intervention–Evaluation) charting was introduced in 1984 at the Craven Regional Medical Center in North Carolina. With this method, problems are identified and addressed at least once on every shift. Teaching plans are incorporated in the progress notes. Notes must be read often to understand the evolution of the problems and the effectiveness of the treatment.

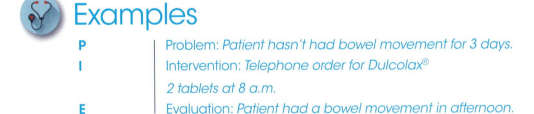

Examples

P	Problem: *Patient hasn't had bowel movement for 3 days.*
I	Intervention: *Telephone order for Dulcolax®* *2 tablets at 8 a.m.*
E	Evaluation: *Patient had a bowel movement in afternoon.*

Whatever system your office or institution follows is the system one needs to utilize for progress note, documentation, patient achievements, charting in the medical record, or the electronic medical record.

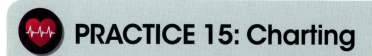 **PRACTICE 15: Charting**

Respond to the following items:

1. An example of subjective information is _____.

   a. giving pain medication   b. a patient's complaint

   c. history of the problem   d. physical therapy

2. Dr. Lawrence Weed developed a medical record system called _____.

   a. HMRO   b. the traditional method

   c. POMR   d. chronological system

3. Which of the following is subjective?

   a. diagnosis   b. treatment

   c. lab report   d. past surgical history

Charting and Documenting Summary

Medical record/chart	Information about a patient's health condition and landmarks in health care.
Language of the medical record/chart	Use medical terms for documenting medical information.
	States have two letter abbreviations—MA, NY.
	Certifications and registrations have no periods—RN, CMT, CMA.
	Measurement abbreviations have no periods.
	A comma is not necessary when II or III follows a surname—John Archie IV.
	In formal writing, days of the week and months of the year are not abbreviated—February 18, 20XX.
Types of charting	
Traditional	Chart notes that use phrases, clauses, and sentences without any specific structure.
Problem Oriented Medical Record (POMR)	Charting problems by order of importance.
SOAP	An acronym meaning:
	S—subjective data: feelings and description of symptoms.
	O—objective data: data from physical exam.
	A—assessment: diagnosis and impressions.
	P—plan: medication, treatments, consults, surgery.

SOAPE	E—evaluation: patient's response to treatment.
SOAPIE	I—intervention: an approach to a particular problem.
	E—evaluating that approach.
SOAPIER	I—intervention: approach to a problem.
	E—evaluating that approach.
	R—revision: changes prompted by the evaluation.
PIE	Problem-Intervention-Evaluation
	Problems are identified and addressed at least once on every shift.

 # Skills Review

Identify the italicized words as a phrase or a clause:

1. Studying is essential *while attending college courses.* _____

2. A pregnant woman can give diseases *to her unborn child.* _____

3. Medical information is kept confidential *unless a release form is signed.* _____

4. Weight varies according to one's exercise patterns. _____

5. *After she completed the form,* she proofread it for errors. _____

6. The journal printed last month had an article *about cancer research.* _____

7. *Although vital signs were stable,* the patient remained in surgical recovery. _____

8. A physician, *with years of experience,* performed the operation. _____

9. *When you know the test results,* give me a call. _____

10. Chris's goal is to do research *in the medical profession.* _____

Underline any phrases within the paragraph:

Education is a vital service to both patients and physicians. Patients often experience anxiety over health concerns. Health care providers must foster patient confidence and trust. The medical assistant tries to establish a rapport between the patient and physician. Medical assistants often suggest to patients that they prepare questions for the doctor.

The assistant may also alert the physician of a patient's health concerns. Information about fees, office hours, insurance, office policies, and Medicare should also be readily available. In this manner, the medical assistant performs a vital service to both patients and physicians. The services of medical assistants are a great value to the medical profession.

Underline any clauses within the paragraph:

Health care providers must educate patients who need specific health information. Patient education is an important function of the allied health professional. When a professional deals with patients, state medical information in clear, concise language that patients can understand. Gathering additional information such as pictures, pamphlets, films, and community resources is also helpful. After completing patient education, evaluate the session's effectiveness. Health care providers who educate patients about health issues provide valuable information that could help the patient throughout life.

Comprehensive Review

Complete these fragmented sentences:

1. For medical coverage to continue. _____
2. Your medical insurance representative. _____
3. The results from your computerized tomography test. _____
4. An adjustment made to the patient's claim. _____
5. People with job-related illnesses. _____

Select the best sentence from among the three choices:

1. A. I see an arrhythmia on the telemetry call the cardiologist.

   B. I see an arrhythmia on the telemetry, call the cardiologist.

   C. I see an arrhythmia on the telemetry. Call the cardiologist.

2.   A. The person is dyspneic, she needs oxygen.

     B. The person is dyspneic; she needs oxygen.

     C. The person is dyspneic she needs oxygen.

3.   A. The biopsy is tomorrow I hope for good news.

     B. The biopsy is tomorrow, therefore, I hope for good news.

     C. The biopsy is tomorrow, and I hope for good news.

4.   A. The hospital wing is closed repairs are being made.

     B. The hospital wing is closed because repairs are being made.

     C. The hospital is closed, repairs are being made.

5.   A. A nurse expresses compassion when she works with her patients.

     B. A nurse expresses compassion when he works with his patients.

     C. Nurses express compassion when they work with their patients.

Improve these sentences. (Many of them were obtained from actual doctor's reports.)

1.   The operation was successful and the patient left the operating room in excellent condition. _____

2.   If you should have any questions or comments please don't hesitate to call me. _____

3.   The patient moved slowly. She moved along the corridor, She used her walker. _____

4.   After the operation, bring the patient to the next room over in the recovery room. _____

5.   The problem was here yesterday and it will be here tomorrow unless you do something about it today. _____

6.   If my secretary has not called you yet, please call her and schedule a 45 minute consultation. _____

7.   This communication is to notify you that your results to your blood chemistry are normal. _____

8.   The patient drinks several beers a day and occasionally a cigar or cigarette. _____

9. Hot compresses to the right hand. _____

10. Hygiene was carefully enforced. _____

Circle the correctly spelled word in each line:

1. chemotherputic	chemotherapeutic	chemotheraputic	chemotherapuetic
2. dihiscence	dehiscence	dehisence	dehissence
3. evisceration	evicseration	evisserration	eviseraetion
4. difusion	diffussion	diffusion	difuesion
5. intoxcication	intoxsication	intoxecation	intoxication
6. narcopsy	narrcolepsy	narkolepsy	narcolepsy
7. dysplasia	dyspaysia	dysplaysia	displasia
8. imunoglobulins	inmunoglobulins	immunoglobulins	immunoglobbulins
9. incontenence	incontinence	incontanence	incontonance
10. asessment	asesment	assessment	assesment

SECTION 7
Punctuation

Practical Writing Component: Medical Reports

Objectives

After reading this section, the learner should be able to:

- use the appropriate punctuation marks at the ends of sentences
- use internal sentence punctuation correctly
- spell various medical terms
- recognize reports: history and physical, consultation

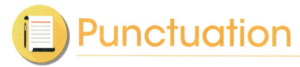

Punctuation

The purpose of *punctuation* is to make the written message easier to read and understand. To understand the importance of punctuation, read the following paragraph out loud:

> *Health care professionals often work in teams a team that is committed to the task and makes full use of its members talents can achieve high levels of performance cooperation is needed for success in a spirit of cooperation people recognize the benefits of helping one another no one person has all the answers but each person has a piece of the puzzle once the pieces are shared the larger picture is clear and possible solutions are easier members need to feel that they are important and that they have something to contribute they claim ownership when they have a share in making decisions carrying out policies or solving problems members must trust and have confidence in one another trust is built when there is an atmosphere of honesty fairness sensitivity and respect a trusting environment helps members to feel comfortable enough to share their talents and reveal their opinions people who benefit most from high quality performance are the patients*

The previous paragraph shows how difficult it is to make sense out of a text when punctuation is missing. Knowing how to use punctuation correctly is an important skill. Doctors who dictate information often do not include punctuation. Punctuation is used for clarity and organization in your writing.

The Period

A period is used at the end of a sentence. It is also used within a sentence as internal punctuation.

 ## Examples

Bradycardia indicates a low pulse. [End of a declarative sentence.]

Follow the doctor's orders. [End of an imperative sentence.]

Schedule an appointment for next week. [End of an imperative sentence.]

Use a period to separate dollars and cents and whole numbers with decimals (decimal point). Do not use a period after whole numbers not accompanied by decimal fractions.

 ## Examples

I paid $16.50 for my scrubs.

The incision was 5.3 centimeters.

My membership fee was $125 a year.

Use a period after most abbreviations.

 ## Examples

Dr. Loveland is the physician on call.

Ms. Martin, please admit Mrs. Arlene Channel.

Jane L. Alexander is Rene's instructor.

Medically related abbreviations may appear in upper or lower case and with or without a period. Do not use periods with measurements.

 ## Examples

The kidney stone measured 5 mm in length.

He was 6 ft tall.

The patient was a 52 yo male.

A period is not placed after state abbreviations, ZIP codes, or acronyms. Acronyms are made up of the first letters in a series of words. They are sometimes pronounced as words.

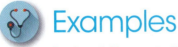 ## Examples

Boston, *MA*	*CA*	*OH*	*CT*	*FL*	Douglas, *MA* 01516
AMA	*AAMA*	*CMA*	*CNA*	*AARP*	*OSHA*

A period follows the letters and numbers in list or outline enumerations.

 ## Examples

1. Nouns
2. Pronouns
3. Verbs

I. Medical Reports
A. History and Physical
B. Pathology
C. Discharge Summary

The Question Mark

A question mark is used after a direct question.

 ## Examples

Where is the pain?

What is the diagnosis?

How much medication was ordered?

Do you know what the cure is for that disease?

"When can I go home?" asked the patient.

The Exclamation Point

Use the exclamation point after a sentence that expresses strong feelings.

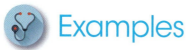 ## Examples

Ouch!

Call security!

Congratulations!

What a wonderful way to stay healthy!

 # PRACTICE 1: End Punctuation

Place the appropriate punctuation marks at the ends of these sentences:

1. The trachea functions as a passageway for air to reach the lungs

2. The symptoms are fever and headache

3. Is pruritus recorded as an objective symptom

4. The portion of the History and Physical where the physician uses hands and fingers during an examination is called palpation

5. The embolus traveled to the lungs

The Comma

Within sentences, the comma is the most frequently used punctuation mark. It is also the punctuation mark that causes the most difficulty. Errors fall into two extreme categories: Commas are either disregarded, or they are used too frequently. The main purpose of the comma is to group words that belong together and separate words that do not. A comma also represents a brief pause when reading. The best rule to follow about commas is not to use it unless there is a reason to do so.

RULE 1: The comma is used to separate three or more items in a series.

 ## Examples

Coryza, cough, and sore throat are common in the winter.

Influenza is characterized by the sudden onset of *chills, headache, and myalgia.*

The five stages of grieving are *denial, anger, bargaining, depression, and acceptance.*

If items in a series are each linked by *and* or *or,* a comma is not used.

 ## Examples

The four blood types are A *and* B *and* AB *and* O.

Martha *and* John *and* Megan are coming to the conference.

RULE 2: Use a comma to separate two or more adjectives that describe the same noun.

 ## Examples

Purulent, rusty-colored sputum was taken to the lab for testing.

The x-ray revealed *numerous, questionable nodules.*

RULE 3: A comma is used between two independent clauses joined by coordinating conjunctions (*and, but, or, nor, for, so, yet*).

 ## Examples

Medicare is administered by the Social Security Administration, *but the public welfare office handles Medicaid.*

Patients usually recover rapidly from influenza, *yet some patients experience lassitude for weeks.*

RULE 4: Place a comma between the day and year. If a date is used in a sentence, a comma goes between the year and the rest of the sentence.

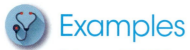

Examples

February 28, 2009

On *February 28, 2009,* the hospital will review its policies.

RULE 5: Use a comma between the city and state. When the city and state are used in a sentence, a comma is placed after the state.

Examples

Boston, Massachusetts

Anesthesia was first discovered in *Boston, Massachusetts,* at Massachusetts General Hospital.

The American Association of Medical Assistants and the American Medical Association are located in *Chicago, IL.*

RULE 6: Use a comma to separate numbers that have four or more digits.

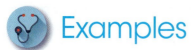

Examples

3,000   30,000   300,000   3,000,000

Exceptions include addresses and year numbers of four digits.

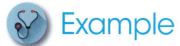

Example

The address is *3600* Main Street.

RULE 7: Use a comma to separate appositives, nouns of direct address, titles that follow a person's name, and introductory words from the rest of the sentence.

Examples

Doctor, please listen carefully to what I have to say.

Please listen carefully, *Doctor,* to what I have to say.

Yes, you may have a regular diet.

However, I do think you will have to curtail your intake of cholesterol.

A decrease in total dietary fat will help, *however.*

Dr. Loveland, *a pathologist,* graduated from a medical school in Burlington, VT.

The pathologist, *Norm Villamarie, M.D.,* graduated from a medical school in Burlington, VT.

RULE 8: Use a comma to separate clauses and phrases that are unnecessary to the meaning of a sentence (nonessential, or nonrestrictive, clauses and phrases).

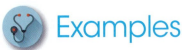

Examples

The hospital, *unlike most facilities,* has a comprehensive evacuation plan.
[*Unlike most facilities* is not necessary to the meaning of the sentence.]

The hourly pay, *in some circumstances,* increases over a period of time.
[The sentence still makes sense when *in some circumstances* is omitted.]

Programs, *which are available on request,* are free of charge.

RULE 9: A comma follows the salutation in a friendly letter and the complementary close.

Examples

Dear Friend, Hello, Suzanne,

Yours truly, Sincerely, Best regards,

RULE 10: Separate parenthetical expressions with a comma, depending on where they are placed in the sentence. Parenthetical expressions include:

I believe (think, hope, see, etc.)		**I am sure**	**on the contrary**
on the other hand	**after all**	**by the way**	**incidentally**
in fact	**indeed**	**naturally**	**of course**
in my opinion	**for example**	**however**	**nonetheless**
to tell the truth			

Examples

The surgery was successful. *Therefore,* there is no need of further treatment.

The report, *I hope,* will give you many options about treatments.

The signs and symptoms, *in my opinion,* are indicative of angina pectoris.

An inadequate supply of oxygen to the myocardium, *for example,* is caused by arteriosclerosis.

RULE 11: Use a comma to separate a direct quotation.

Examples

The doctor said, *"You must give up smoking."*

"I really don't have the courage," the patient replied.

"In that case," the doctor continued, *"you sign your own death warrant."*

RULE 12: A comma is used to set off contrasting statements that are introduced by the words *not, rather,* and *though*.

Examples

Right now, *rather* than later, increase the medication.

I would describe her mood as thoughtful, *not* sullen.

PRACTICE 2: Commas

Punctuate these sentences:

1. The divisions of the vertebrae are cervical thoracic lumbar sacral and coccygeal

2. A tickler file is a reference system of call-back appointment dates and future events

3. Prior to antibiotics her sinusitis caused headaches

4. The symptoms are vomiting drowsiness shock pallor diaphoresis and liver tenderness

5. The patient is instructed to wash the skin avoid scrubbing and keep hands away from the face

6. I don't believe it

7. The patient replied "I don't want my family to know"

8. Is there a history of myocardial infarctions in the family

9. After July 15 send my mail to Albany NY 02863

10. Someday I will work as a Certified Medical Assistant in the doctor's office

The Semicolon

The semicolon is a punctuation mark that is stronger than a comma; that is, it indicates a more definite break in the flow of a sentence. Semicolons join items that are grammatically alike or closely related.

RULE 1: A semicolon is used instead of a comma and a coordinating conjunction (*and, but, or, nor, for, yet, so*) to separate two independent clauses.

 ## Examples

The physician shall respect the law; he shall recognize the responsibility to change any law that is contrary to the best interest of the patient.

Almost all victims of violence go to emergency centers; many have no health insurance.

Many people are homeless because they were discharged from a mental institution; most are without proper follow-up health care.

If a coordinating conjunction is present, commas are used to separate independent clauses. The clauses can also be rewritten as two sentences.

Examples

The cost of health care in the United States is out of control; 37 million have no health insurance and 35 million are underinsured.

The cost of health care in the United States is out of control; yet 37 million have no health insurance and 35 million are underinsured.

The cost of health care in the United States is out of control. Thirty-seven million have no health insurance and thirty-five million are underinsured.

RULE 2: Use a semicolon between independent clauses when the second clause begins with a transitional expression such as:

for example	*for instance*	*otherwise*
that is	*besides*	*therefore*
accordingly	*moreover*	*consequently*
nevertheless	*furthermore*	*however*
instead	*hence*	*namely*

 # Examples

Every medical office has its unique pathology format; *however,* the data required is the same.

The arterial blood gas reports are good; *therefore,* we can begin the process of weaning from the ventilator.

The cardiac rate was rapid and regular; *consequently,* there are no extrasystoles.

The patient was afebrile after admission; *nevertheless,* he became febrile with recurrent episodes of pain in the left side of the chest.

Note: A comma sets off one independent clause: "*The medical report is completed,* all ten pages." A semicolon sets off two independent clauses: "The medical report is completed; mail it first class."

RULE 3: Use a semicolon with a series of items that have one or more commas.

 # Examples

Those present at the meeting were Dr. Loveland, my family physician; Mrs. P. Archibald, my lawyer; Jake, my husband; and Valerie, my daughter.

I sent copies to Miami, Florida; Albany, New York; and Boston, Massachusetts.

 ## PRACTICE 3: Semicolons

Punctuate these sentences:

1. I wanted a response from Dr. Villamarie a forensic pathologist from Boston but as of today I have received none

2. Call Dr. Flemming the surgeon Kim Yonta the lawyer and Chris Browning the medical insurance representative

3. Valerie visited the medical library on Tuesday she also did further research on Saturday

4. The importance of determining the comparability of the two drug groups is evident for example eleven deaths are due to surgery five to acute myocardial infarction and six to embolic complications

5. Some redness pain and swelling appeared in the right ankle consequently ice packs were applied

The Colon

The colon is a sign that more information follows. The information may be expressed in a series of words, phrases, or clauses.

RULE 1: A colon is used to introduce a list or series of items.

 Examples

The pathology report consists of the following: the patient's name, medical record number, tissues submitted, findings, impressions, and possible treatment.

The only explanations I can give are these: the patient didn't follow directions, forgot to take the medication, or stopped taking it because of side effects.

I made a list of the things we need: forceps, 4–0 catgut sutures, gauze sponges, and surgical scissors.

I made a list of the things we need:

1. forceps
2. 4–0 catgut sutures
3. gauze sponges
4. surgical scissors

RULE 2: A colon is not used if a verb or preposition immediately precedes a series of items. Whatever precedes a colon should be a complete sentence.

 Examples

The health team consists *of* physicians, nurses, a physical therapist, and a nurse aide. [preposition]

We *need* forceps, 4–0 catgut sutures, gauze sponges, and suture scissors. [verb]

RULE 3: A colon is used between hours and minutes to express time.

 Examples

6:15   8:30 a.m.   8 a.m. (Do not use zeros for on-the-hour time.)

RULE 4: A colon is used in business letters.

 Examples

Dear Dr. Archibald:

To Whom It May Concern:

Re: Medical Report #1234235

C: President Macgilvery

Christopher Ramirez

PRACTICE 4: The Colon

Punctuate these sentences:

1. SOCIAL HISTORY The patient neither smokes nor drinks

2. Is my appointment at 11 30 or 1 30

3. Many medical assistants were at the Cancer Conference Chris Luke John Valerie and Sarah

4. Tissues involved

    1. Node from the left lung

    2. Right mediastinal nodes

    3. Carina

    4. Left lung

5. Discharge diagnoses

    A. Excision of benign cyst of left lung

    B. Emphysema

    C. Klebsiella pneumoniae infection

6. Fibrous tissue extending out from the vitreous was covered with many vessels

7. To Whom It May Concern

8. Digitalis therapy was begun because of dyspnea chest pain and swelling of the legs

9. The cases were arterial insufficiency diabetes gangrene glomerulonephritis and anemia

10. Marked interstitial edema was present with diffuse mononuclear infiltrate composed of lymphocytes and plasma

Parentheses

RULE 1: Parentheses surround information that is added but unnecessary and unrelated to the main thought of the sentence.

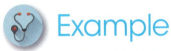

Example

The nurses from the second floor (*Lisa, Kurt, Nancy, and Ramon*) make a great team.

RULE 2: Parentheses are used around an abbreviation or acronym that follows the spelled out version, or vice versa.

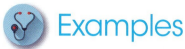 Examples

The medical assistant (*MA*) is responsible for typing the report.

OSHA (*Occupational Health and Safety Association*) provides valuation information to hospitals.

RULE 3: Use parentheses around numerals or italic letters that designate enumerations of list items within a sentence.

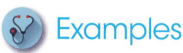 Examples

The instructions are (*a*) more fluids, (*b*) aspirin 2 tabs whenever necessary, and (*c*) bedrest.

The instructions are (1) more fluids, (2) aspirin 2 tabs whenever necessary, and (3) bedrest.

The Dash

The purpose of the dash (—) is to set off unnecessary items from the rest of the sentence. The reason for using the dash, rather than any other punctuation mark, is to give more emphasis to words. The dash may be applied singly or in pairs. However, it is rarely seen in medical documentation.

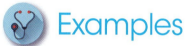 Examples

I have 30 years—*very rewarding ones*—of medical practice.

The forms are to be written exclusively by physicians—*not nurses, not therapists, not social workers, and not aides.*

The Hyphen

The hyphen is also covered in Section 4, under "Predicate and Compound Adjectives." Because punctuation is so important in medical documentation, a short introduction is included here.

RULE 1: Use a hyphen between compound words used as an adjective when the adjective precedes the noun.

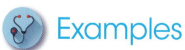 Examples

| *all-day* surgery | *102-year-old* man | *grayish-black* tissue |
| *follow-up* | *one-by-one* | |

A *well-developed, well-nourished* young man.

A *34-year-old* male was admitted to the West Wing.

When a compound modifier follows the noun, it is not hyphenated.

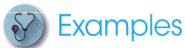 Examples

The young man was *well developed.*

Compound words that have become commonly used are not hyphenated.

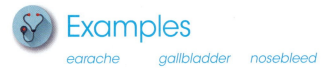 Examples

earache   *gallbladder*   *nosebleed*

RULE 2: Use a hyphen with numbers 21 to 99 and with written fractions.

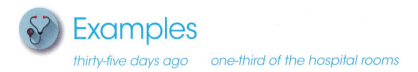 Examples

thirty-five days ago   one-third of the hospital rooms

RULE 3: Use a hyphen with a prefix added to a word that begins with a capital letter.

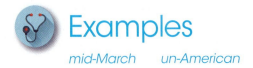 Examples

mid-March   un-American

RULE 4: Some adjective forms are always hyphenated, whether before or after the nouns they modify.

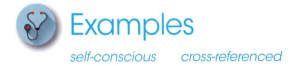 Examples

self-conscious   cross-referenced

RULE 5: Use a hyphen in some compound words used as nouns.

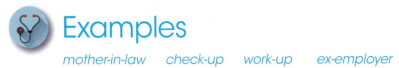 Examples

mother-in-law   check-up   work-up   ex-employer

Always consult the dictionary when in doubt about hyphenation.

The Apostrophe

Another punctuation mark often used in medical reporting is the apostrophe. An apostrophe is used to show ownership (referred to as the possessive form of a noun).

Please refer to the chapter on nouns.

Italics

Italic print is used for emphasis, words used as terms, or words used as words. If italic print is not available, underlining is used.

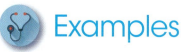 **Examples**

All surgical equipment *must* be sterilized before use.

The term *officious* could be applied to his tone in the letter.

Friendly and *polite* are not synonymous.

Italics are also used in the following instances:

- Titles of books, magazines, and newspapers

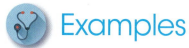 **Examples**

New England Journal of Medicine

New York Times   Gray's Anatomy

Lancet   *Taber's Cyclopedic Medical Dictionary*

Harvard Health Letter   *JAMA*

- Movies, television, radio, plays, and operas

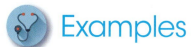 **Examples**

Mozart's Requiem

Did you watch *ER* on television last night?

- Foreign expressions

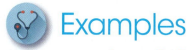 **Examples**

mea culpa: my fault

fait accompli: carried out with success

respondeat superior: "Let the master answer."

res ipsa loquitur: "Let the thing speak for itself."

- All biological names

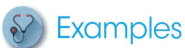 **Examples**

Clostridium difficile   Staphylococcus aureus

Streptococcus pyogenes   *Escherichia coli*

Pseudomonas aeruginosa   *Salmonella enteritidis*

Haemophilus influenza   *Campylobacter jejuni*

Quotation Marks

Quotation marks are used to enclose the exact words of the speaker. Quotations are often used when it is necessary to quote the exact words of the patient or a family member.

 ## Examples

Claudia said, "*I have pain in my chest.*" [The period goes inside the quotation mark.]

"*I go to physical therapy at 3 p.m.,*" said Sheila. [The comma goes inside the quotation mark.]

"*Take the patient to room 205,*" Robert said, "*while I bring the chart to the desk.*" [Note the interruption of the quotation.]

"*What was the hematocrit?*" asked Dr. Matthews. [Note the question mark inside the quotation mark.]

"*I would advise caution,*" said the physician, "*because your condition is serious.*" [Note the interruption of the quotation.]

Quotation marks are also used to enclose a part of a completed published work or to indicate that words or phrases are being used in a special way.

 ## Examples

Chapter 9 is titled "Punctuation."

The title of the seminar is "Stress Management."

Write "confidential" on the envelope.

 ## PRACTICE 5: All the Rest

Punctuate these sentences:

1. The chapter entitled Punctuation is the most important chapter in the book.
2. Quick said John get the defibrillator!
3. We got the article out of the New England Journal of Medicine.
4. The vertebrae are composed of thirty three bony segments.
5. Yogurt is a form of curdled milk caused by Lactobacillus bulgaricus.
6. The preoperative medication is due forty five minutes before surgery.
7. The side effects of the medication are 1 headaches 2 possible vomiting and 3 diarrhea.
8. The speaker was very self conscious.
9. Yellow fever is caused by the bite of the female mosquito Aedes aegypti.
10. JAMA and the Lancet published the study.

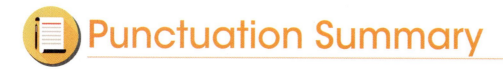

Punctuation Summary

Period*

After a statement	You looked better after your treatments.
With abbreviations	Dr. R. Williams │ a.m. │ $50
Not with abbreviations of measurements	3.5 mm │ ft │ gal

Question Mark*

After a question	At what time is the operation scheduled?
	How old were you on your last birthday?

Exclamation Point*

After an exclamatory sentence	Your house is on fire!
	Get help in here right away!

*The period, question mark, and exclamation point are referred to as end punctuation because they come at the ends of sentences.

Comma:

Used to group words that belong together, separate words that do not belong together, and provide a brief pause.

In a series	The recovery rooms are painted in aqua, light blue, lavender, and white.
Between two adjectives before a noun	A confidant, trustworthy nurse is hard to find.
	I'm looking for an inexpensive, comfortable car.
Before *and, but, or, nor, yet* following an independent clause	I have good medical coverage, but it expires when I leave my job.
Around unnecessary clauses and phrases	Computers, used correctly, can save time. To the best of my knowledge, the situation no longer exists.
	Looking ahead, we can prepare for the event.
Following introductory elements	Well, we can do it again to make sure.
Around parenthetical expressions	In fact, I did pass with honors.
Around appositives	If you believe that, John, you can believe anything.

Other uses

Following the salutation of a friendly letter	Dear Mom,
Following a complimentary close	Sincerely yours,
Between city and state	Chicago, Illinois 68594
Between date and year	October 11, 20XX
To separate quotations	"I came by car," replied the salesman.
In numbers of four or more digits	600,000
Preceding a title after a person's name	Dr. Judith Powers, Ph.D.

Semicolon:

Used to indicate a more definite break than a comma in the flow of a sentence and to join items that are grammatically alike or closely related.

Between independent clauses not joined by a coordinating conjunction *(and, but, or)*	I saw red; I was so angry.
Between independent clauses joined by *however, hence, that is, therefore,* etc.	Computers are faster; therefore, use them for scheduling appointments.

Separating elements in a series that contain commas	Cities and countries participating are Rome, Italy; London, England; and Ottawa, Canada.

Colon:

Used to indicate that more information is coming.

Preceding a series, list, or outline that is introduced by a complete sentence.	Consider the following: less expensive, better quality, and good returns on investment.
Between minutes and hours in expressions of time	9:15 p.m.
Following the salutation of a business letter	Dear Mr. President:

Parentheses:

Used to mark off explanations.

Around added information unrelated to the main thought	The physicians (all eight of them) donated services to the needy.
Around words added to clarify the sentence	The AMA (American Medical Association) is a powerful organization.
Around numbers or letters that designate enumerations of list items within a sentence	The best things to do are (1) take a fever reducer, (2) get plenty of rest, and (3) drink a lot of fluids.

Dash:

Used to set off unnecessary items from the rest of the sentence.

Adds emphasis	She won the prize—a trip to Disney World.

Hyphen:

Used between elements of compound words or numbers and to divide words into syllables.

Compound words, syllables	state-of-the-art equipment
With written numbers 21 to 99	twenty-five years ago
In written fractions	one-half the population
Between a prefix and the base word	un-American
	self-explanatory

Apostrophe:

Used to show ownership.

Forms the possessive	Singular: patient's disease, boss's policy
	Plural: patients' diseases, bosses' policies

Italics:

Used in place of an underline to point out or emphasize.

For names of books, magazines, works of art, biological names, foreign expressions	I subscribe to the *PMA*.
	E. coli is normal flora in the G.I. tract.

Quotation Marks:

Used to enclose the exact words of a speaker.

Around a direct quotation	The doctor said, "Be sure to take your medication."
Around all segments of an interrupted quotation	"Be sure to take your medicine," said the doctor, "or you won't get well."
Around parts of published works	The article "The Pathology of Germs" can be found on the Internet.
Around words or phrases used in a special way	The president's diagnosis was so "confidential" that even reporters weren't aware of it.

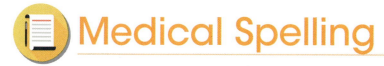

Medical Spelling

Become familiar with the spelling of the following words:

afebrile	embolus	myalgia	Salmonella
anesthesia	febrile	myocardium	Staphylococcus
angina	filtration	neuromuscular	Streptococcus
arteriosclerosis	forceps	nodules	tracheostomy
buccal	hematology	norepinephrine	thrombus
cholesterol	infiltrate	opaque	ventilate
curette	insufficiency	papilla	vitreous
defibrillator	interstitial	penicillin	well-developed
digitalis	Kaposi's sarcoma	percussion	well-nourished
earache	keratitis	purulent	Xylocaine

Real-World Applications

Punctuation marks (. ? ! , ; : ' " ") can either clarify or confuse the meaning of a sentence or abbreviation. To misplace one of these small but important symbols can create confusion or frustration for the reader; just think of what might happen if your bank misplaced a comma or decimal point in your account records!

For this reason, punctuation marks must be given special attention in all forms of medical writing. Medical reports, such as a history and physical report, are just one example of medical writing in which punctuation is key to understanding.

Medical Reports

History and Physical Reports

A *history and physical (H&P) report* is usually dictated after a new patient is admitted to a hospital or comes to a clinic, office, or health facility. The H&P is a collection of data about past events in relation to a patient's present illness (Figure 7-1). Its purpose is to aid in understanding the whole patient, past and present, in order to form a treatment plan based on how the patient can be helped in the future.

The format of the report varies from place to place and is usually generated by the medical facility's Form Committee. Regardless of the format, however, the type of information sought is universal.

The historical component is an account of the patient's systems and organs based on information rooted in the past, such as family and social histories, previous hospitalizations or treatments, allergies, chronic illness, and the patient's chief complaints. The physical component of the H&P is not historical. It is the physician's current evaluation of the patient's systems and organs.

HISTORY AND PHYSICAL EXAMINATION (H&P)

Patient Name: Roger Parks

Hospital No.: 11009

Room No.: 812

Date of Admission: 12/01/20XX

Admitting Physician: Steven Benard, M.D.

Admitting Diagnosis: Rule out appendicitis.

CHIEF COMPLAINT: Abdominal pain.

HISTORY OF PRESENT ILLNESS: The patient is a 31-year-old white man with acute onset of right lower quadrant pain waking him up from sleep at approximately 3 a.m. on the morning of admission. The pain worsened throughout the day, radiating to his back and becoming associated with dry heaves. The patient states that the pain is constant and is worsened by walking or movement. The patient states his last bowel movement was on the previous evening and was normal. The patient is anorectic. He also gives a 1-year history of lower abdominal colicky pain associated with diarrhea. He was seen by his local medical doctor and given a diagnosis of irritable bowel syndrome; however, the pain is worse tonight and is unlike his previous bouts of abdominal pain. The patient also has had associated fever and chills to date.

PAST HISTORY: SURGICAL: No previous operations.

ILLNESSES: None. Hospitalization for epididymitis 10 years ago. He is ALLERGIC TO PENICILLIN. It makes him bloated.

MEDICATIONS: None.

SOCIAL HISTORY: Carpenter. Lives with his wife and two children. He does not drink or smoke.

FAMILY HISTORY: Insignificant for familial inflammatory bowel disease except for the fact that his mother has colonic polyps. Father living and well. No siblings.

REVIEW OF SYSTEMS: Noncontributory.

PHYSICAL EXAMINATION: This is a 31-year-old white man with knees raised to his abdomen and complaining of severe pain. VITAL SIGNS: Admission temperature 99.6F; four hours after admission it was 102.6F. HEENT: Normocephalic, atraumatic, EOMs intact, negative icterus, conjunctivae pink. NECK: Supple. No adenopathy or bruits noted. CHEST: Clear to auscultation and percussion. CARDIAC: Regular rate and rhythm. No murmurs noted. Peripheral pulses 2+ and symmetrical. ABDOMEN: Bowel sounds initially positive but diminished. He has positive cough reflex, positive heel tap, and positive rebound tenderness. The pain is definitely worse in his RLQ. RECTAL: Heme negative. Tenderness toward the RLQ. Normal prostate. Normal male genitalia. EXTREMITIES: No clubbing, cyanosis, or edema. NEUROLOGIC: Nonfocal.

LABORATORY DATA: Hemoglobin 14.6, hematocrit 43.6, and 13,000 WBCs. Sodium 138, potassium 3.8, chloride 105, CO_2 24, BUN 10, creatinine 0.9, and glucose 102. Amylase was 30. UA

FIGURE 7-1 Sample History & Physical Report

M.A. Novak and P.A. Ireland, *Hillcrest Medical Center Beginning Medical Transcription Course*, 6th ed. Albany, NY: Delmar Thomson Learning, 2005, pp. 16–17.

completely negative. LFTs within normal limits. Alkaline phosphatase 78, GGT 9, SGOT 39, GPT 12, bilirubin 0.9. Flat plate and upright films of the abdomen revealed localized abnormal gas pattern in right lower quadrant. No evidence of free air.

ASSESSMENT: Rule out appendicitis. Some concern of whether this could be an exacerbation of developing inflammatory bowel disease. Due to the patient's history, increasing temperature, and localizing symptoms to his right lower quadrant, the patient needs surgical intervention to rule out appendicitis.

_____

Steven Benard, M.D.

SB:xx

D:12/01/20XX

T:12/01/20XX

FIGURE 7-1 Continued

Consultation Report

When a consultation has been requested to obtain a second opinion on a problem or diagnosis, a *consultation report* is prepared for the referring physician. It contains such data as present medical history, x-ray and lab results, and the consulted physician's impressions, recommendations, evaluations, diagnoses, and treatment (Figure 7-2).

Promptness in providing information is very important. The consultation report format may be a letter or a specially prepared form with the date and reason for consultation.

It is also proper to include a thank you for the referral. The report is dictated by the consulting physician and transcribed in the medical office or through outside services.

 # Medical Reports Summary

History and Physical	A report containing data about past events in relation to a patient's present illness.
Consultation	A report containing data such as present medical history x-ray lab results, consulted physician's impressions, recommendations, evaluations, diagnoses, and treatments.

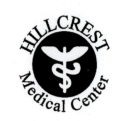

REQUEST FOR CONSULTATION

Patient Name: Marty Gibbs

Hospital No.: 11532

Consultant: Patrick O'Neill, M.D., Plastic Surgery

Requesting Physician: Diane Houston, M.D., Internal Medicine

Date: 11/25/20XX

Reason for Consultation: Please evaluate extent of burn injuries.

BURNING AGENT: Coals in fire pit.

I have been asked to see this 5-year-old Caucasian male who appears in mild distress due to upper extremity burn after having fallen into hot coals in his back yard.

Using the Lund Browder chart,[4] the severity of burn is first and second degree. The total body surface area burned includes right lower arm 3%, right hand 1%. The joints involved include the right elbow, right wrist, right hand.

TREATMENT PLAN: Splinting right hand.

                       Positioning: Elevation with splint on.

                       Range of motion: Good mobility.

                       Pressure therapy: Will follow for induration, for pressure fracture.

GOALS:
1. Reduce risk of contractures of involved joints by positioning, splinting, and maintaining range of motion.
2. Reduce scar tissue formation by using Jobst bandages, pressure therapy, and splinting.
3. Obtain maximum mobility and strength of upper extremities.
4. Maximize independence in activities of daily living. Activity as tolerated.
5. Provide patient and family education regarding high-calorie, high-protein diet.

Thank you for asking me to see this delightful boy. I will follow him at the burn clinic in 2 weeks.

_____

Patrick O'Neill, M.D.

PO:xx

D:11/25/20XX

T:11/28/20XX

[4]See page 221: The Lund Browder Chart.

FIGURE 7-2 Sample Consultation Report

M.A. Novak and P.A. Ireland, *Hillcrest Medical Center Beginning Medical Transcription Course,* 6th ed. Albany, NY: Delmar Thomson Learning, 2005, pp. 21–22.

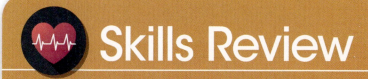

Skills Review

Punctuate these sentences if necessary:

1. Because new drugs are pure chemicals they are dispensed by weight

2. Four common routes of antibiotic are intravenous intramuscular oral and local

3. If you do not receive your raise by the first of the year be sure to inform the personnel department

4. Objects should never be placed inside a cast to relieve itching relief comes by applying a cold pack over the cast where the itch is located

5. A patient is instructed on how to care for the cast limit activities use devices such as crutches or a cane and perform prescribed exercises

6. Coryza is a general term for a cold or inflammation of the respiratory mucous membranes

7. Over the counter medications are available for cough headache and fever

8. The large intestines are about 1.5 m long and are divided into 4 parts the ascending the transverse the descending and the sigmoid colon

9. Diabetes meaning *passing through* is a general term for excessive urination and is usually referred to as diabetes mellitus

10. ADMITTING DIAGNOSIS Rule out cholecystitis cholelithiasis

Punctuate and capitalize these sentences:

Health care professionals often work in teams a team committed to the task makes full use of its members talents and can achieve high levels of performance cooperation is needed for success in a spirit of cooperation people recognize the benefits of helping one another no one person has all the answers but each person has a piece of the puzzle once the pieces are shared the larger picture is clear and possible solutions are easier members need to feel that they are important and that they have something to contribute they claim ownership when they have a share in making decisions carrying out policies or solving problems members must trust and have confidence in one another trust is built when there is an atmosphere of honesty fairness sensitivity and respect a trusting environment helps members to feel comfortable enough to share their talents and reveal their opinions people who benefit most from high quality performance are the patients.

Use "H&P" (history and physical) or "C" (consultation) to answer each statement:

1. Usually requested to obtain a second opinion. _____

2. Dictated after a patient is admitted for a surgical procedure. _____

3. Prepared for the referring physician. _____

4. Current evaluation of the patient's systems and organs. _____

5. Specific knowledge about a system of the body. _____

Circle the correctly spelled word in each line:

1. ceratitis   keratitis   karatitis   kerratitis

2. kolesterol   cholisterol   cholesterol   cholestirol

3. interstitiol   interstichial   interstiel   interstitial

4. myalgia   mialgia   myalgea   myolgia

5. artiriosclerosis arteriscelrosis arteriosclerosis arterioclerosis

6. Strepcoccus   Stretcocucus   Steptococcus   Streptococcus

7. bukkal   bucal   buccal   buccle

8. insuficiency   insufficiency   insifficency   insphiciency

9. Xylocaine   Xylocane   Xylicaine   Zylocaine

10. pencillin   penicillin   penecillin   pinicilin

 # Comprehensive Review

Rewrite, type, and punctuate the following paragraphs:

John miller a 31 year old adult came into the office of dr beth winters on February 12 20XX at 815 complaining of acute abdominal pains the pains were exacerbated by any type of body movement the patient has a long history associated with diarrhea a condition diagnosed as irritable bowel syndrome the patient said the pain was unlike any previous troubles of abdominal pain

_____

_____

_____

_____

_____

_____

_____

_____

_____

_____

a physical examination showed these factors 102° temperature and no adenopathy or bruits noted bowel sounds were initially positive but diminished films reveal localized ab-normal gas pattern in the right lower quadrant

_____

_____

_____

_____

_____

_____

_____

_____

_____

SECTION 8
Prepositions, Conjunctions, and Paragraphs

Practical Writing Component: Research Manuscripts

Objectives

After reading this section, the learner should be able to:

- recognize prepositions, compound prepositions, and prepositional phrases
- use prepositional phrases as modifiers
- understand problematic prepositions
- recognize coordinating, correlative, and subordinating conjunctions
- spell various medical terms
- recognize paragraphs
- understand research for manuscripts and promotional writing used in the medical profession

Prepositions

A *preposition* shows how a noun or pronoun is related to another word or group of words in a sentence. It is a connective word that joins a noun or pronoun to the rest of the sentence. Prepositions are used very often in speaking and writing. A prepositional phrase is nonessential and can be removed entirely from a sentence.

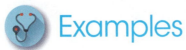

Examples

Sociology is the study *of* the origins *of* society.

Anatomy is the science *of* the structure *of* the body and the relationship *of* its parts.

"Physio-" refers *to* nature. Physiology is the study *of* the functions and activities *of* the living body.

Radiopaque means impenetrable *to* x-rays. X-rays do not go *through* metals.

Dr. Jack and Dr. Jill went *up* the hall *to* fetch a liter *of* intravenous fluid.

Dr. Jack fell *down* the hall and broke his arm. Dr. Jill came tumbling *after* him.

The words in italics, the prepositions, show the relationship to the nouns and pronouns in the sentences.

Some prepositions help to show location or place: *between, below, near, on, against, in,* and *through.*

Examples

Lateral is situated away *from* the midline *of* the body.

Intercostal is *between* the ribs.

Subcostal means *below* a rib.

Decline means *to* go down *to* something lower.

Dorsal means *toward* or situated *on* the back side.

The medical report is *on* the table.

In the anatomical position, the body is facing forward *with* the arms *at* the sides and the palms *toward* the front.

A few prepositions show a relationship of time: *before, during, since,* and *until.*

Examples

Before performing the examination, wash your hands carefully.

The intern fell asleep *during* the lecture.

I can't pay my medical loans *until* I get a job.

During the delivery of the Rh-positive baby, some of the baby's blood cells containing antigens may escape *into* the mother's bloodstream.

Other prepositions show different kinds of relationships between a noun or pronoun and another word: *about, among, by, for, from, like, of, to,* and *with.*

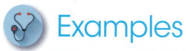

Examples

Rh immune globulin is given *to* the mother *to* help prevent the antigen-antibody reaction.

Antibiotics inhibit the growth *of* microorganisms.

Biopsy is the examination *of* tissue *from* the body.

The biopsy was taken *from* the lymph node.

A professional relationship exists *among* doctors and health care professionals.

Some prepositions indicate direction: *around, beside, under, through, across, over, toward,* and *to.*

Examples

The sterile drape was placed *over* the Mayo stand.

The cast is molded *around* the contours of the body.

Place the tourniquet *around* the arm three or four inches *above* the venipuncture site.

The physical therapist put the patient *through* range of motion exercises.

Common Prepositions		
about	between	on/onto
above	beyond	out/outside
across	by	over
after	concerning	past
against	despite	round
along	down	regarding
amid	during	since
among	except	through, throughout
around	for	till
as	from	to, toward
at	in/into	under, underneath
before	inside/outside	until
behind	like	unto
below	near	up/upon
beneath	of	with/without/within
beside/besides	off	

Compound Prepositions

Compound prepositions are groups of two or three words that are used so frequently together that they function like one-word prepositions.

Commonly Used Compound Prepositions

according to	in addition to	in terms of
along with	in back of	in support of
apart from	in connection with	next to
as for	in contrast to	on account of
as regards	in defense of	on behalf of
as to	in front of	out of
aside from	in place of	together with
because of	in reference to	with reference to
by way of	in regard to	with regard to
contrary to	in spite of	with respect to
due to	instead of	

As a word of caution regarding compound prepositions, avoid using two or three words when a single word will suffice.

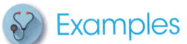

Examples

Compound	Place the patient's medication *next to* the file.
Singular	Place the patient's medication *beside* the file.
Compound	Medical supplies are kept *inside of* the cabinet.
Singular	Medical supplies are kept *in* the cabinet.
Compound	Rose is doing well *in spite of* her sickness.
Singular	Rose is doing well *despite* her sickness.
Compound	Rubber gloves are placed *down under* the shelf.
Singular	Rubber gloves are placed *under* the shelf.
Compound	Medical assistants' uniforms are made *out of* synthetic materials.
Singular	Medical assistants' uniforms are made *of* synthetic materials.

PRACTICE 1: Compound Prepositions

Underline the compound preposition and its object:

1. According to the physician, the patient can exercise in spite of his injury.
2. Because of the cancer metastasis, the patient will be discharged.
3. Dr. Villes spoke in support of the consultation.
4. I thank you on behalf of my staff for your dedicated service.
5. With respect to the involved personnel, this has been a team effort.

Prepositional Phrases

A *prepositional phrase* begins with a preposition and ends with a noun or pronoun that is its object.

 ## Examples

by next Wednesday	under the fascia
through the bloodstream	for the patient
at work	regarding the long-term prognosis

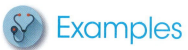 ## PRACTICE 2: Prepositional Phrases

Underline the prepositional phrases:

1. Throughout the exam, Mrs. Griffs was very cooperative and without pain.

2. The liver removes bilirubin from the blood.

3. Vitamin K aids in the clotting of blood and is responsible for the production of prothrombin.

4. Vitamin D aids in the building of bones and the body's use of calcium and phosphorus.

5. The normal pulse rate for toddlers and very young children is 80 to 100 pulsations per minute.

Prepositional Noun/Pronoun Modifiers

A *prepositional noun/pronoun modifier* is a prepositional phrase that is used to modify a noun or pronoun. Such phrases are usually found in one of two positions: after the word being modified or after a linking verb.

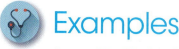 ## Examples

An *assistant* to the doctor made the travel arrangements to the conference.

The purpose of splinting prevents *motion* of the injured part.

The medical *report* is on the table.

He *is* in the waiting room.

PRACTICE 3: Prepositional Noun Modifiers

Underline the prepositional phrase, and circle the noun it modifies:

1. An insurance company charges a premium for its coverage.

2. A patient with emphysema uses the Fowler's position.

3. The autoclave in the treatment room is working.

4. All employees in the medical office must observe asepsis.

5. Hypertension is a major contributor to heart attacks.

Prepositional Verb Modifiers

Prepositional verb modifiers are prepositional phrases that modify verbs and answer the questions *how? when? where?* and *to what extent?*

 ## Examples

The tricuspid valve is located *in the heart.* [where?]

The medication must be taken *with meals.* [when?]

The surgeon dictates the surgical procedure *in great detail.* [to what extent?]

Prepositional phrases that modify verbs can occupy different positions in the sentence, thus enabling the writer to emphasize different points.

 ## Examples

At last, the patient agreed to undergo treatment.

The patient agreed *at last* to undergo treatment.

The patient agreed to undergo treatment *at last.*

Good writing focuses on the reader rather than the writer. Starting a sentence with the word *I* can easily be avoided by beginning the sentence with a prepositional phrase instead.

 ## Examples

On Friday, I spoke to the x-ray technician.

In spite of the work involved, I want to write the article for the medical journal.

PRACTICE 4: Prepositional Verb Modifiers

Underline the prepositional phrase, and circle the verb it modifies:

1. Personality remains stable during normal aging.

2. Repression occurs when painful thoughts are forced into the unconscious.

3. Tissues that are removed in surgery are sent to pathology.

4. Illness is denied through defense mechanisms.

5. Viruses live within other cells and can be seen only by electron microscopes.

Circle all of the prepositions in this paragraph:

"I will follow that system of regimen which, according to my ability and judgment, I consider for the benefit of my patients, and abstain from whatever is deleterious and mischievous. I will give no deadly medicine to anyone if asked, nor suggest any such counsel; and in like manner I will not give to a woman a pessary to produce abortion. With purity and with holiness I will pass my life and practice my art. I will not cut persons laboring under the stone, but will leave this to be done by men who are practitioners of the work. Into whatever houses I enter, I will go into them for the benefit of the sick, and I will abstain from every voluntary act of mischief and corruption; and, further, from the seduction of females or males, of freemen and slaves. Whatever, in connection with my professional practice, or not in connection with it, I see or hear, in the life of men, which ought not to be spoken of abroad, I will not divulge, as reckoning that all such should be kept secret." (Taken from the Hippocratic Oath)

Problematic Prepositions

Prepositions that often cause difficulty in writing are *between* and *among,* and *beside* and *besides. Between* refers to two people, things, or groups and *among* refers to more than two:

Information *between* a patient and a physician is highly confidential.

Among all the students in the class, she was the one who worked in the OR.

Beside means "next to" and besides means "in addition to" or "except":

The oxygen tank is *beside* the bed.

There is another insurance company *besides* that HMO that offers the benefits;

PRACTICE 5: Between, Among, Beside, Besides

Identify the correct word within parentheses:

1. (Beside, Besides) radiation, the patient must also have chemotherapy.
2. This information is shared (among, between) the doctor and the patient.
3. The medication was placed (beside, besides) the glass of water.
4. Hospital physicians are (among, between) the personnel who attended the meeting.
5. Corridors (between, among) the first and second floor must be locked.

Other prepositions that often are misused are *to, different from, in,* and *into.* The problem with the preposition *to* is that it sounds like the words *two* and *too. To* is a preposition meaning toward something, *two* is a number and a noun, and *too* is an adverb meaning "also."

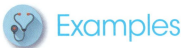

Examples

John went *to* the science lab.

Two opinions are needed by the insurance company.

I'd like more medical information, *too.*

Confusion exists about the use of the preposition *from* after the word *different.* The preferred expression is *different from* rather than *different than.*

Examples

Use *different from* when it means the same as "differs from something else."
[The recommendation was *different from* ours.]

Use *different than* with the comparative degree of adjectives and adverbs.
[Mr. Jones's training was *different than* Mr. Smith's.]

The preposition *in* refers to a location or movement within an area:

The file is *in* Dr. Villes' office.

The preposition *into* means "entry, introduction, insertion, superposition, or inclusion":

The doctor and lawyer entered *into* a mutual agreement, and then the patient came *into* the conference room.

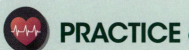

PRACTICE 6: In, Into, To, Different

Identify the correct word to be used from within the parentheses:

1. The supervisor wanted the nurse to look (in, into) the causes of the injury.
2. A heart operation is very (different than, different from) a lung operation.
3. Medical personnel entered (in, into) a discussion about cancer treatment.
4. Isopropyl alcohol is used to clean the surface of the skin, (to, too, two).
5. Put the specimen (in, into) the container.

Prepositions at the End of a Sentence

Many English instructors maintain that a sentence ending with a preposition is weak. However, it is an acceptable practice to do so in certain situations, such as when the preposition is part of the previous verb and when the end preposition emphasizes a strong point.

 ## Examples

I am sending you some reports to look *at*. Read them *through*.

The medical team can be counted *on*.

The side effects were too much to contend *with*.

Where did the cancer metastasize *from*?

In formal writing, it is best to try to place the preposition anywhere but at the end or to rewrite (but without being awkward).

 ## Examples

Medicare is for patients 65 years of age or *over*.

Medicare is for patients *over* 65 years of age. (better)

The subject of death and dying is difficult to talk *about*.

Death and dying is a difficult subject *about* which to talk. (awkward)

Chris is the person I work *with*.

I work *with* Chris. (better)

What is the book *about*?

The book is *about* what? (awkward)

Where is this medication shipped *to*?

Where is the medication shipped? (better)

PRACTICE 7: Placement of Prepositions

Rearrange the preposition within the sentence or otherwise revise for clarity:

1. These symptoms are something I never heard *of*. _____

2. Cathy feels it necessary to drain the water *off*. _____

3. I changed the dressing *after* physical therapy. _____

4. What are you in the hospital *for*? _____

5. The anesthesiologist put the patient *under*? _____

Conjunctions

A *conjunction* is another part of speech that joins words or parts of sentences. There are three types: co-ordinating, correlative, and subordinating.

Coordinating Conjunctions

The coordinating conjunctions *and, but, or,* and *yet* are used to join two single words or groups of words of the same kind or of equal construction.

Examples

Dr. Hebert *and* Dr. Balin prepared for surgery. [The conjunction *and* joins two proper nouns, *Dr. Hebert* and *Dr. Balin,* to form a compound subject.]

Ask Kate *or* Jane to cover the main desk. [The word *or* connects or joins the two indirect objects, *Kate* and *Jane.*]

His speech was short *but* effective. [*But* connects the equal construction of the two predicate adjectives, *short* and *effective.*]

She said she'd be late, *yet* she arrived on time. [*Yet* connects the group of words relating the similar constructions, *she'd be late* and *she arrived on time.*]

Correlative Conjunctions

Correlative conjunctions consist of two elements used as pairs to connect parallel structures.

both … and	*Both* the doctor *and* the nurse were present.
not only … but also	The machine *not only* copies materials *but also* sorts.
either … or	*Either* I *or* my assistant will be in the ER.
whether … or	I'm going *whether* you are *or* you're not.
neither … nor	*Neither* the doctor *nor* the nurse could contain the patient on the stretcher.

Subordinating Conjunctions

The subordinating conjunction begins an adverb clause and joins the clause to the sentence. This type of conjunction is covered in detail in the section on sentences.

PRACTICE 8: Conjunctions

 PRACTICE 8: Conjunctions

Identify the conjunction and state whether it is coordinating or correlative:

1. Give Valerie or Christopher a call at the hospital. _____
2. Both chemotherapy and radiation are needed for this type of cancer. _____
3. Runny nose and general malaise are symptoms of a cold. _____
4. You can make a dental appointment either now or later. _____
5. Either set the fracture now or bring the patient for a CT scan. _____

Prepositions and Conjunctions Summary

Prepositions	Shows how a noun/pronoun is related to another word or group of words in a sentence; a connective word that joins a noun/pronoun to the rest of the sentence: "The letter continues *on the next page.*"	
Compound prepositions	Two to three words that function like one preposition.	I'm calling *in regard to* the package I received *by way of* Federal Express.
Prepositional phrases	Begins with a preposition and ends with a noun or pronoun that is its object.	The procedure took place *in the operating room.*
Prepositional modifiers:		
Noun/pronoun modifiers	Found after the word modified or after a linking verb.	The reason *for the meeting* is obvious. The reports are filed *under the letter S.*
Verb modifiers	Modifies a verb and answers *how? when? where?* and *to what extent?*	The answer is found *in the last chapter.* (where)
		The medication is taken *before going to bed.* (when)
Problematic prepositions	Between—refers to two.	This information is just *between* us.
	Among—refers to more than two.	Patience is listed *among* the qualities.

	Beside—next to.	Stand *beside* me during the announcement.
	Besides—in addition to.	*Besides* the book there is a map.
	To—the preposition.	Go *to* the OR STAT!
	Two—the number.	*Two* problems exist in the report.
	Too—also.	I'm going, *too*.
	Different from is the preferred expression over different than.	This treatment is *different from* the last one.
Prepositions at the end of a sentence	An acceptable practice when preposition is part of a previous verb or emphasizes a strong point. Try to avoid it at the end in formal writing.	This is one thing you have to attend *to*.

Conjunctions

Joins words or parts of sentences

Coordinating	Joins two single words or groups of words of the same kind or equal construction: and, but, yet.	"Vitamin D is found in liver, butter, *and* green vegetables." "The wound is healing, *yet* it still needs to be covered."

Correlative

Pairs of words used to connect parallel structures:

	both . . . and:	"*Both* Ben *and* his wife are sick."
	not only . . . but also:	"The doctor is *not only* a surgeon *but also* an instructor."
	either . . . or:	"The patient comes in *either* today *or* sometime next week."
	whether . . . or:	"*Whether* the scrubs are green *or* yellow is up to you."
	neither . . . nor:	"*Neither* the x-ray *nor* other tests revealed any problem."
Subordinating	Begins an adverb clause and joins it to the sentence.	"*Before* she left the doctor's office, she paid her copayment."

Summary of the Parts of Speech

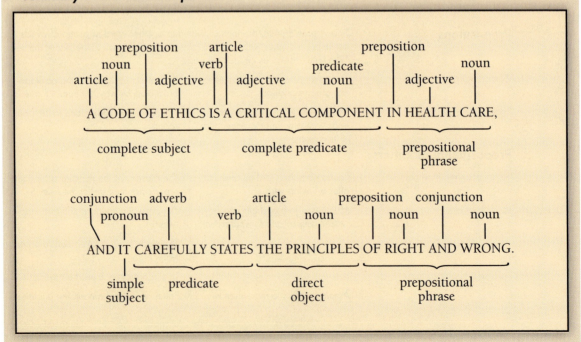

FIGURE 8-1 Summary of Parts of Speech

Medical Spelling

Become familiar with the spelling of the following words:

antiemetic	electrode	manipulation	sanitization
antihistamines	eliminated	metastasis	semi-Fowler's
asepsis	fascia	nausea	specimen
asphyxia	flatulence	palpitation	sterilization
autoclave	Fowler's position	percussion	syncope
bilirubin	fumigation	postprandial	technique
cyanotic	hazardous	prothrombin	Trendelenburg
deficiency	hypertension	pruritus	urticaria
diaphoresis	isopropyl	regime	vertigo
diaphragm	lithotomy	regimen	viruses

Paragraphs

Ultimately you want to deliver an effective message. A message that contains sentences that are related. Sentences creating unity and coherence in paragraph form. A *paragraph* is a group of sentences that go together because they explain a common point of view called a *main idea.* A main idea is the central message that the writer wishes to convey to the reader. That message is what drives the entire passage. Every sentence in an effective paragraph must be related to the main idea. A paragraph is easy to detect because the start of its first sentence is indented about five spaces from the left-hand margin. The length of a paragraph varies, depending on the complexity of the main idea.

 PRACTICE 9: Paragraphs

PRACTICE 9: Paragraphs

All three of the following paragraphs give the same message. Which one is easiest to read and understand?

1. The doctor's office is more than a professional health care service. It is also a business. Because of this reality, an efficient system of record management is needed to maintain a well-directed medical office practice. The first component of medical records deals with a patient's health information. Data include such items as a medical history examination results, record of treatments, laboratory reports, prescriptions, and diagnoses. Invoices, insurance forms and policies, payroll records, canceled checks, financial records, and other correspondence pertain to the business component of the operation. More than likely, business information is filed separately from a patient's health record. Medical professionals may draw on four or five different filing methods to maintain order: alphabetic, numeric, geographic, subject, and color-coding. Efficient record management is essential for the smooth operation of both components of a medical office practice.

2. The doctor's office is more than a professional health care service. It is also a business. Because of this reality, an efficient system of record management is needed to maintain a well-directed medical office practice.

The first component of medical records deals with a patient's health information. Data include such items as a medical history, examination results, record of treatments, laboratory reports, prescriptions, and diagnoses. Invoices, insurance forms and policies, payroll records, canceled checks, financial records, and other general correspondence pertain to the business component of the operation.

More than likely, business information is filed separately from a patient's health record. Medical professionals may draw on four or five different filing methods to maintain order: alphabetic, numeric, geographic, subject, and color-coding. Efficient record management is essential for the smooth operation of both segments of a medical office practice.

3. The doctor's office is more than a professional health care service. It is also a business. Because of this reality, an efficient system of record management is needed to maintain a well-directed medical office practice.

The first component of medical records deals with a patient's health information.

Data include such items as a medical history, examination results, record of treatments, laboratory reports, prescriptions, and diagnoses.

Invoices, insurance forms and policies, payroll records, canceled checks, financial records, and other general correspondence pertain to the business component of the operation.

More than likely, business information is filed separately from a patient's health report.

Medical professionals may draw on four or five different filing methods to maintain order: alphabetic, numeric, geographic, subject, and color-coding.

Efficient record management is essential for the smooth operation of both components of a medical office practice.

 # PRACTICE 10: Forming Paragraphs

Separate this message into three paragraphs:

Patients often wonder why the social history (SH) component is part of medical records. On further investigation into the meaning of social history, the reason becomes evident. Habits of smoking, physical exercises, eating, sleeping, and hobbies greatly impact the health of every individual. Facts about a patient's family history provide the physician with additional health data. Hereditary factors and parent and sibling health conditions help doctors see the larger picture. Questions on the review of symptoms (ROS) concentrate on the patient's general health condition unrelated to the present illness. The ROS provides a history of systems and organs, usually in logical order from head to foot.

_____

_____

Types of Paragraphs

Many different types of paragraphs exist. The four types most commonly encountered by people in the medical profession are narrative, descriptive, expository, and persuasive.

Narrative Paragraph

As the term implies, a *narrative paragraph* tells a story or shows a series of events that usually occur in chronological order. Narrative paragraphs may be autobiographical (about oneself), biographical (about another), or about something witnessed.

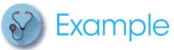 **Example**

Elizabeth Blackwell, an immigrant from England, was the first woman in the United States to receive a degree in medicine. She was refused entrance into medical school many times before she was finally accepted. While practicing in this country, she established a hospital staffed by women. Returning to England, she founded the London School of Medicine for Women.

Descriptive Paragraph

A *descriptive paragraph* is a pictorial representation in words that appears in most types of writing. The choice of words in this type of paragraph is deliberately specific to describe concrete details about objects, ideas, actions, settings, or persons. The wording conveys a sensory impression of appearance, smell, taste, sound, and touch or reveals a mood or an emotion.

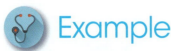

Example

The professor in the anatomy lab described the heart in the following manner:

The heart is a muscular organ located between the lungs. It weighs about nine ounces and is about the size of a fist. The heart has four chambers. The two upper chambers, the atria, are the receiving chambers and the two lower chambers, the ventricles, are the pumping chambers. Valves are located between the upper and lower chambers that open and close to let the flow of blood pass in one direction.

Expository Paragraph

An *expository paragraph* is the most common type of paragraph. Its purpose is to inform, explain, or define something. The information may include facts, statistics, or specific examples. Because the language is so precise, the tone of the paragraph is very factual and unemotional.

Example

The patient's chief complaint is headache pain on one side of the head. If this is a migraine, it exhibits certain characteristics. Migraines have a high hereditary influence and commonly affect more women than men. The usual symptoms are severe, intense, and of long duration. It often presents when the person wakes in the morning. One side of the head is affected more than the other. The pain may be more severe over the temporal area but also may include the face and other areas of the head. Other signs and symptoms that may occur at the attack are nausea and/or vomiting, fatigue, irritability, chilliness, edema, diaphoresis, or aphasia.

Persuasive Paragraph

The *persuasive paragraph* is written to urge the reader to follow a certain course of action, to deal with an important issue, or to state an opinion about a debatable issue. The topic sentence clearly and concisely states the writer's point of view. Subsequent sentences develop the issue with reasonable and supportive statements.

Example

One critical pathway for increasing the effectiveness of medical care in hospitals is to adopt quality assurance standards. These standards encompass every facet of the hospital from medical personnel, patients, staff, and administration. Other components include medical care, patients' rights, family satisfaction, hospital policies, cost-effectiveness, and medical records. The Joint Commission establishes quality assurance standards. The implementation of these standards is a necessity if growth is to take place in the health care industry.

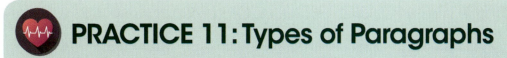

PRACTICE 11:Types of Paragraphs

Identify this paragraph as descriptive, expository, or persuasive:

Electrolytes are chemical compounds found in all body fluids. Electrolytes break into positive and negative particles that conduct electrical impulses. Acids, bases, and salts are examples of electrolytes. Some general functions of all electrolytes are (1) to promote neuromuscular irritability, (2) to maintain body fluid volume, (3) to distribute water between fluid compartments, and (4) to help regulate the acid-base balance. Electrolytes are a necessity for life.

Structure of a Paragraph

The structure of the paragraph consists of three elements: the topic sentence, supporting sentences, and a concluding sentence. The topic sentence presents the main idea. Subsequent supporting sentences offer more details about the topic. The concluding sentence brings closure to the paragraph (Figure 8-2).

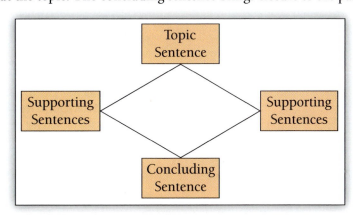

FIGURE 8-2 The Structure of an Effective Paragraph

Topic Sentence

The topic sentence is the most important sentence in the paragraph because it introduces the reader to the main idea. It tells the reader what the paragraph is about and helps keep ideas organized and focused. In a sense, the paragraph is a clear and direct summary of the main idea. A paragraph without a topic sentence misdirects and confuses the reader. The topic sentence should immediately capture the interest of the reader.

Supporting Sentences

The supporting sentences form the body of the paragraph and comprise the details, facts, examples, descriptions, definitions, explanations, questions, causes and effects, comparisons, contrasts, and proofs that support the main idea expressed in the topic sentence. The more specific the details of the supporting sentences, the better the explanation of the main idea. The content of the body usually answers any number of questions like *who? what? what kind? where? when? why?* and *how?*

Concluding Sentence

The final sentence brings the paragraph to a conclusion in one of several ways. It may summarize, offer a solution, predict, make a recommendation, state a conclusion, or restate the topic sentence.

Putting the Paragraph Together

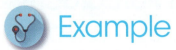

Example

Topic Sentence	Punctuation is a crucial skill for medical assistants to possess.
Supporting Sentences	Many physicians do not bother to punctuate their reports, letters, notes, or correspondence. Should punctuation be included, it is often used incorrectly. The end punctuation of sentences is usually correct because the punctuation marks are obvious. The punctuation mark that causes the most problems, however, is the comma. There are more rules for the use of the comma than any other type of punctuation.
Concluding Sentence	Knowing where to place commas is a crucial step in acquiring punctuation skills.
The Complete Paragraph	Punctuation is a crucial skill for medical assistants to possess. Many physicians do not bother to punctuate their reports, letters, notes, or correspondence. Should punctuation be included, it is often used incorrectly. The end punctuation of sentences is usually correct because the punctuation marks are obvious. The punctuation mark that causes the most problems, however, is the comma. There are more rules for the use of the comma than any other type of punctuation. Knowing where to place commas is a crucial step in acquiring punctuation skills.

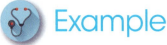

Example

Topic Sentence	An operative note is one type of medical documentation.
Supporting Sentences	This report, dictated by the surgeon or an assistant, describes a surgical operation. The report includes pre- and postoperative diagnoses, sponge count, and blood loss.
Concluding Sentence	The report concludes with the patient's condition at the end of the surgical procedure.
The Complete Paragraph	An operative note is one type of medical documentation. The report, dictated by the surgeon or an assistant, describes a surgical operation. The report includes pre- and postoperative diagnoses, sponge count, and blood loss. The report concludes with the patient's condition at the end of the surgical procedure.

PRACTICE 12: Paragraph Structure

Identify the topic, supporting, and concluding sentences in each paragraph:

1. The rate of respiration may be normal, rapid, or slow. The average rate for an adult is 12 to 20 cycles per minute. The average for infants is 30 to 60. For children age one to seven, the rate is 18 to 30 cycles per minute. The number per minute is referred to as the rate of respiration. Medical office workers should be aware of these facts.

2. Gerontology is the study of the aging process. During this process, the chemical composition of the body changes. Among these changes are a decrease in lean body mass and an increase in vulnerability to different diseases. Stress is also an important factor in aging. Stress decreases cardiac output and brain function. As a result, the aging population is more susceptible to infections and accidents.

3. The electrocardiogram (EKG or ECG) is a recorded picture of the electrical activity of the heart. The EKG may be normal even in the presence of heart disease. It is essential that the EKG be used in conjunction with the patient history, physical exam, and laboratory data. Arrhythmia and dysrhythmia are used interchangeably to denote an abnormal conduction. Electrocardiograms are a necessary component in assessing cardiovascular disease.

4. Communication consists of many types. The spoken word or verbal communication is not the only one. Sometimes people communicate more with actions than with words. A smile or frown, eye contact or lack of it, gestures, postures, touch, and style of dress are expressions of nonverbal communication. In these cases, actions may speak louder than words.

5. Fats, proteins, carbohydrates, vitamins, and minerals are all necessary nutrients for the body. A person's basal metabolic rate, growth, and physical activity determine the amount of nutrients needed. Nutrition needs change when a person is ill, is taking medications, or has a type of trauma. An imbalance occurs when nutrients are consumed in concentrated forms and reach the point that they do not help. Proper nutrition is important to everyone's health.

Paragraph Organization

Paragraphs should be well organized in that the arrangement of their sentences should follow some order. One common way to organize a paragraph is by time. Other ways to organize paragraphs are location, deduction, induction, cause and effect, comparison, and definition or classification.

Time is a chronological approach that lists events from the earliest to the most recent, or in reverse, from the most recent to the earliest. An example of time is a paragraph describing events from 1989 to 2010; a resume is an example of reverse chronological order.

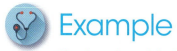 # Example

The American Medical Association, AMA, was organized in 1846 in New York City. A Code of Ethics was formulated and adopted in 1847. Its principles were revised in 1906, 1912, and 1949. In 1957, they were condensed to a preamble and ten sections.

Organizing paragraphs by time, however, is not conducive to documenting ideas. To write about ideas, you should organize the paragraphs by logic. Paragraphs organized by logic proceed from the familiar to the less familiar, simple points to more complex points, less important things to more important things and the general to the specific.

The location approach involves the arrangement of content from left to right, right to left, top to bottom, edge to center, and the like.

 Example

Chart notes are dictated in a SOAP format. *S* refers to *subjective* or what the patient tells the doctor. The *O* for *objective* consists of what the physician finds on examination. *A* is the *assessment* the physician makes or the diagnosis. *P* stands for the *planned* course of treatment.

Organizing by deduction starts with the general and goes to the specific. The topic sentence, which is general, is followed with specific reasons, examples, facts, and details that support the topic sentence.

 Example

Follow these general rules regarding word contractions in medical transcription. Contractions may be used in informal records like chart notes. However, in formal correspondence like reports, use the words that form the contraction (do not, is not) rather than the contractions (don't, isn't).

Induction is the opposite of deduction. Specific ideas come before the general. Details, reasons, and examples follow the topic sentence.

 Example

Letters to insurance companies and physicians are a few examples of correspondence dictated by specialists. To this list may be added follow-up letters concerning referred patients and letters of introduction. Medical office correspondence consists of many different types.

Cause and effect paragraphs help connect the result of something with the events or facts that precede it.

 Example

Prilosec stops the production of stomach acid. It can turn off stomach acid production within an hour. The medication is used for conditions in which stomach acid is produced as part of a condition. Some of the drug's side effects are headache, diarrhea, nausea, fever, and vomiting.

The comparison paragraph measures one subject against another subject. The comparison is presented early. Contrasted details are given to illustrate the differences between the subjects.

Example

Legal abuses that affect health care are physical abuse and verbal abuse. Examples of physical abuse are performing the wrong treatment, hitting, holding the patient too roughly, or failing to answer the call light. Verbal abuse is using profanity or raising a voice in anger. Failure to obey laws regarding abuse results in fines or imprisonment.

Paragraphs organized by definition or classification explain words and ideas in a clear fashion.

 ## Example

Pulse, respiration, temperature, and blood pressure are called vital signs. Pulse is the regular throbbing of the arteries echoing contractions of the heart. Respiration is the process of breathing and is measured by watching a patient breath in and out. Temperature is the degree of heat within the body. Blood pressure is the amount of force exerted by the heart pumping blood through the arteries. Vital signs are extremely important because appropriate medical care depends on these readings.

PRACTICE 13: Organization of Paragraphs

Identify the following paragraphs as organized by time, location, deduction, induction, cause and effect, comparison, definition, or classification:

1. *Advice* is a noun that means an opinion or a recommendation: My *advice* to you is to get a second opinion. *Advise* is a verb that means to inform or to recommend: I would *advise* you to get a second opinion. _____

2. When arranging flight reservations for the medical conference, obtain departure date and time, flight number, and estimated time of arrival. Make hotel reservations and arrange transportation from the airport to the hotel in time for the conference. The same information is required for the return trip: transportation to the airport, departure and arrival times, and arrangements for the traveller to be picked up at the airport and driven home. _____

3. Alzheimer's disease is caused by changes in nerve endings and brain cells that interfere with normal brain function. Symptoms of Alzheimer's progress from simple forgetfulness to severe loss of memory about how to dress, eat, or call people by name. Other signs are unpredictable moods and personality changes. _____

4. *Effect* is a noun that means the result of some action: A side *effect* of antihistamine is sleepiness. *Affect* is usually a verb that means to impress or influence, usually in the mind or feelings: The death of the patient *affected* us. _____

5. Locating a file on the computer is likened to locating a file in a file cabinet. Entering the A or C drive on the computer is similar to opening a drawer of the file cabinet. Clicking the subdirectory on the computer (A:\Dr. Villes\consults) is comparable to opening a file pulled from the drawer. _____

Paragraph Unity

In addition to structure and organization, an effective paragraph should also have unity. Unity means that sentences should flow logically from one statement to another. Ideas are arranged and connected so they will read smoothly and sensibly. Paragraph unity is achieved in a number of ways, one of which is called *transition*. A transition is a word, phrase, or structural element that appropriately links one sentence to the next by referring to previously used words or ideas:

> *Bathing* is as important to the sick as it is to persons who are well. *Besides* removing dirt and perspiration, *bathing* helps patients relax.

Examples of transitional words are *finally, consequently, also, thus, in another sense, in the same way, specifically, nevertheless, nonetheless, besides, on the other hand, above, below, meanwhile, moreover, however, as I said above, still, therefore, furthermore, in addition, similarly, in contrast, on the contrary, for example, accordingly, as a result, consequently, next, yet, that is, in particular, at last, likewise, more important, then, in summary, on the whole, as a matter of fact, during, after, before,* and *the first point.*

Transitional words can be grouped by location, time, comparison, contrast, emphasis, summary, additional information, or clarity:

Location	*across, around, away from, beyond, in back of over, outside*
Time	*while, first, during, next, as soon as, finally, till, at, after*
Comparison	*in the same way, likewise, also, similarly*
Contrast	*although, on the other hand, yet, however*
Emphasis	*to repeat, in fact, for this reason, again*
Summary	*as a result, therefore, in conclusion, to sum up, all in all*
More information	*additionally, besides, for instance, likewise, along with*
Clarity	*in other words, for instance, that is, put another way*

Other ways to unify a paragraph include these strategies:

- Repeating words from one sentence to the next:
  - The patient was *examined* in the emergency room. On *examination,* the patient's chest and lungs sounded relatively clear.
  - The medical history contained many *errors.* An incorrect spelling of the patient's surname was one of the major *errors.*
- Using pronouns that refer to a noun in a previous sentence:
  - *The nurse instructor* insisted that her students use *medical abbreviations* correctly. *She* gave the class a test on *them* daily.
- Repeating a sentence structure:
  - *A diagnostic report describes* the pathological findings of a sample of tissue. The *MRI uses* electromagnetic energy to produce images of body tissue.
- Substituting another word in place of a previous one:
  - The *Hb, Hct, WBC,* and *RBC* are normal. The *complete blood count (CBC)* is normal.

- Stating at the beginning of a sentence that there are a particular number of points to be mentioned:

  - According to Dr. Elizabeth Kubler-Ross, patients facing death pass through *five* stages. *The first* stage is denial and *the second* is anger.

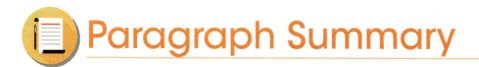

Paragraph Summary

Types of Paragraphs

Narrative	Relates a story or series of events, usually in chronological order.
Descriptive	Describes details, ideas, actions, settings, or persons.
Expository	Informs, explains, or defines something.
Persuasive	Urges the reader to follow a certain course of action, deal with an issue, or state an opinion about a debatable issue.

Paragraph Structure

Topic sentence	Introduces the reader to the main idea.
Supporting sentences	Comprise the details, facts, examples, and questions that support the topic sentence.
Concluding sentence	Brings the paragraph to conclusion.

Paragraph Organization   ## The orderly arrangement of sentences.

Time	Organizes by time.
Location	Arranges from left to right, top to bottom, and edge to center.
Deduction	Starts with the general and goes to the specific.
Induction	Starts with specific and goes to the general.
Cause and effect	Connects results of something to an event or fact.
Comparison	Measures one subject against another subject.
Definition	Explains words or ideas in clear fashion.

Paragraph Unity   ## Methods:

The manner in which sentences are formed smoothly, sensibly, and logically.

- —Repeat words from one sentence to another.
- —Use pronouns that refer back to another noun.
- —Repeat sentence structure.
- —Substitute new words in place of previous ones.
- —Use transition words.

Medical Spelling

Become familiar with the spelling of the following words:

affect	defuse	infraction	petal
Alzheimer's disease	diffuse	keratosis	profusion
arrhythmia	effect	ketosis	reflex
aural	elicit	moral	reflux
cite	explicit	morale	sight
coarse	facial	oral	somatic
complement	fascial	osteopenia	vesical
compliment	illicit	ostalgia	vesicle
course	implicit	pedal	waive
cytology	infarction	perfusion	wave

Real-World Applications

Medical Writing

The diversity of writings in the medical profession is vast, ranging from a single one-page information sheet to a research paper containing multiple pages. Some types of medical writings are listed below:

Medical Journals:	Articles written for the public or the lay person in simple language.
Medical Education:	Written for medical and scientific professionals. New knowledge and material that is written for patients' education.
Publications:	Journal articles for conferences and medical or scientific meetings.
Promotional Writing:	Medical-related writing that may include patient advocacy materials, posters, brochures, announcements, informational material, newsletters, patient education, or other types of important information.
Research Paper:	An investigation into a topic to obtain facts or theories.

Manuscripts and Research

Research is the activity of obtaining information about a subject. It involves such skills as planning, critical thinking, reading studies, and interviews. Often it involves researching literature, publications, and dissemination of facts. Medical assistants are routinely responsible for the mechanics, editing, and organization of multiple pages of data.

APA Writing Style

Term papers, research papers, empirical studies, literature reviews, theoretical articles, methodology articles, and case studies should follow the American Psychological Association (APA) style of scientific writing. It was developed by behavioral and social scientists to standardize writing styles. A copy of *The Publication Manual of the American Psychological Association* can be obtained from: www.apastyle.org /products/index.aspx.

Consider these basic APA guidelines for *manuscript* structure:

- Title page
- Abstract
- Introduction
- Method
- Results
- Discussion
- References
- Appendices

Formatting the paper is discussed in the manual. Some general guidelines include:

- Use a serif font/typeface as Times New Roman for the text.
- Double space the entire manuscript.
- Double space the reference list and figure captions.
- Indent the first line of every paragraph one half inch.
- Align the text to the left margin, with ragged edge at the right margin.
- Submitting the manuscript means the pages would have to be numbered consecutively.
- Title page would be page 1. Abstract page would be page 2. The introduction of the text would begin on page 3.
- References begin on a new page.
- The appendix begins on a new page.

Headings are important because they are the key points to your paper and the evolution of your thoughts. There are five levels of headings in the APA style (Figure 8-3). Some tips for writing headings include:

- Use heading levels in consecutive order.
- Be specific with your writing when relevant.
- Be sensitive to labels, knowing that they change over times.

1. **Center, bold, upper and lower case**
2. **Flush to the left, bold**
3. **Indented, bold, lower case paragraph heading with a period**
4. ***Indented, bold, italicized, lower case paragraph with a period***
5. *Indented, italicized, lower case paragraph heading ending with a period.*

FIGURE 8-3 Five Levels of Headings in APA Style

Promotional Writing

In addition to the more structured types of writing contained in reports, research papers, and manuscripts, medical-related writing includes *promotional writing* such as advertisements, press releases, announcements, brochures, and informational materials.

Medical facilities publish promotional items in brochures, newspapers, medical journals, and publications (Figure 8-4). Data included in those items may cover any of the following:

- Philosophy
- Description of office practice
- Laboratory services
- Policy on appointments and cancellations
- Medical associations
- Policy of prescription renewal

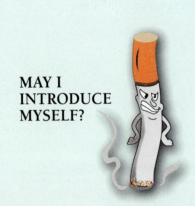

TEEN SMOKE-OUT SEMINARS
October 4, 20XX
January 18, 20XX
March 11, 20XX
May 13, 20XX

**MAY I
INTRODUCE
MYSELF?**

A COLLABORATION
between
VILLES MEDICAL CENTER
and
BARRY HIGH SCHOOL

SPONSORED BY A GRANT
from the
DAVIS FOUNDATION

**I AM A
CIGARETTE!!**

I come in many sizes and shapes, wrapped in shiny, colorful packages that are hard to resist. Advertising agencies show the public how beautiful I am, how "real cool" it is to smoke me, and how wonderful it is to be my friend. Their words flatter me:

Fashionable!

Your basic truth!

You got what it takes!

Enjoy the best of life!

You've come a long way, Baby!

Be the one with STYLE!

You can do it!

Easygoing!

Sleek!

I'm very popular. People in every walk of life respect and hold me in high esteem:

✱ I go to the best of parties.

✱ I'm the first thing people reach for in the morning and the last thing before going to bed.

✱ My friends even leave their homes in the middle of the night to find and smoke me. Spouses and children don't get that much attention.

Others look for me in trash cans or on the street so they can have just one more puff. So what if they get a little dirty. I'm worth it!

I'm also good. The large tobacco corporations that make me provide jobs for thousands of people. From the money you spend, I contribute millions and millions of tax dollars to the world economy. You don't feel that cost when you buy me one pack or one carton at a time. So what if over a 25-year friendship, I cost you the price of a few cars or a college degree. Friends don't let money come between them.

Like everybody else, I'm not perfect. I occasionally burn holes in clothes, rugs, and furniture, causing small fires and injuries.

What really excites me, however, are the homes I burn. The flames make such a pretty sight! Some of these fires claim the lives of my friends, but I don't worry. I'm an arsonist who can't be arrested.

I also cause bad breath, yellow teeth, hacking cough, shortness of breath, heart disease, high medical bills, and even cancer. You could die by associating with me. But don't worry, these things only happen to other people. If you should die, however, your children will give me the pleasure of their friendship by following in your footsteps.

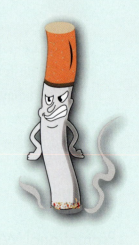

FIGURE 8-4 Sample Brochure

- Map of how to get to the facility
- Parking facilities
- Financial policies
- Photo or logo of the facility
- Names of key medical and administrative staff
- Information for patients prior to their first visit
- Emergency room procedures
- Answering service
- Areas of specialization

Information sheets are a convenient way to distribute data relating to health issues (Figure 8-5). A simple format includes these parts:

- Introduction
- Broad Topic/Narrow Topic

Introduction	Smoking is one of the most overpracticed addictions in the world. Most people who smoke admit that it severely injures their health, but they cannot always explain how. This information sheet briefly relates some reasons why smoking is harmful and why it should be stopped at all costs.
Broad topic	Smoking
Narrow topic	Dangers of not smoking; benefits of not smoking
Points developed	Contents of a cigarette; how a cigarette works in the body; rewards of not smoking
Body, Paragraph 1	
Topic Support	Tobacco wrapped in paper for the purpose of smoking is a lethal weapon. A cigarette is made up of thousands of different chemicals including ammonia (cleaning fluid), nicotine (insecticide), formaldehyde (embalming fluid), arsenic (poison), carbon monoxide (car exhaust), and methanol (wood alcohol). Why do people smoke when they know these chemicals are harmful?
Transition	Consider how nicotine works in the body.
Paragraph 2	
Topic Support	Nicotine hits the brain and makes the smoker feel relaxed and pleasant. The inhaled smoke carries nicotine into the lungs. The blood in the lungs carries the nicotine into the heart and brain—all within seven seconds! Nicotine passes quickly and easily through the entire body in three days. It leaves the bloodstream through the kidneys. If nicotine from ten cigarettes could get trapped in the bloodstream, it would be strong enough to kill a person.
Conclusion	Each year, smoking kills more people than AIDS, alcohol, drug abuse, car crashes, murder, suicide, and fire combined.
Transition	Consequently, people have much to gain by not smoking.
Paragraph 3	
Topic Support	When people quit smoking, their energy improves, they breathe better, the heart works easier, pulse rate and blood pressure become lower, and body circulation improves. The risk of heart attacks and cancer lessens by 90%. More oxygen goes to the brain and the rest of the body, and the sense of taste and smell improves.
Conclusion	In other words, the person gets a second chance at a quality life.
Summary	Cigarettes contain chemicals harmful to the body, even though those chemicals make a person feel "high." More people die from smoke-related illnesses than alcohol, drugs, murder, and suicide combined. After quitting, the risk of a heart attack and cancer is reduced by 90%, thus providing former smokers with a new lease on life.

FIGURE 8-5 Sample Information Sheet

- Points Developed/Subtopics
- Body
- Paragraph 1
- Topic Support
- Conclusion
- Transitional Sentence
- (The same format is used for additional paragraphs.)
- Conclusion
- Summary
- Ending Sentence

Information sheets are used as a handout.

PRACTICE 14: Promotional Writing

Answer true or false whether information in the statements can be included in promotional writing.

1. Name of medical associations. _____

2. Patient's health condition. _____

3. Parking facilities. _____

4. Information from the medical record. _____

5. Financial policies. _____

6. Events that occurred during a patient's stay in the hospital. _____

7. Name of key medical and administrative staff. _____

8. Medical research date. _____

9. Emergency room procedures. _____

10. Correspondence between physicians. _____

Research, Manuscripts, and Promotional Writing Summary

Research	Resources
Investigation into a topic to discover facts and theories.	Medical libraries, the Internet, medical periodicals, public health departments, health care organizations, hospital and clinics, interviews with medical personnel, computer technology software, and clinical studies

Manuscripts	**Type of Content**
Title Page	Title, author(s), affiliations, submission date, for whom written
Abstract	100–150 word summary
Introduction	Problem under study, background, purpose, rationale
Methods	How the study was conducted, procedure
Results	Tables and figures, statistics
Discussion	Evaluation and interpretation of results
Other experiments	Integration of results
References	Supportive interpretations
Appendix	Supplementary materials

Promotional Writing	**Promotional Items**
Formal notice to announce a product or event, provides information, call attention to, or offer goods or services	Brochures, newspapers, medical journals, and publications, advertisements, news releases, and information sheets

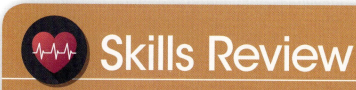

Skills Review

Match these words to the statements listed below:

a. persuasive   **d. deduction**   **g. topic sentence**

b. induction   **e. expository**   **h. comparison**

c. supportive sentence   **f. cause and effect**

_____ 1. Introduces reader to the main idea.

_____ 2. Informs, explains, or defines something.

_____ 3. Starts with the specific and goes to the general.

_____ 4. Starts with the general and goes to the specific.

_____ 5. Connects results of something to an event or fact.

_____ 6. Measures one subject against another subject.

_____ 7. States an opinion about a debatable issue.

_____ 8. Details, facts, and examples that build on the topic sentence.

Divide this passage into appropriate paragraphs.

Many patterns of nursing care are being used today. In the functional method of organizing care, each nursing employee is assigned specific duties to be carried out on all patients in a given unit. For example, a nurse's aide might be assigned to take all the patients' temperatures and the practical nurse to take all the patients' blood pressures. In primary nursing, the nurse is responsible for planning and caring for patients until they leave the hospital. One of the advantages of this pattern is that the nurse is able to give more individualized care. Progressive patient care groups the patients according to degrees of illness, including the patients on the following units: intensive care, intermediate care, self care, long-term care and home care. When the specialized care pattern is used, the patients are grouped according to age or diagnoses. Examples include orthopedics, pediatrics, obstetrics, or geriatrics.

Circle the prepositions in the following paragraph:

John Doe is a 23-year-old male suffering from back pain and memory loss as a result of injuries sustained in a car accident three months ago. At that time, the patient was the driver of an automobile traveling across Main to State Street. Another vehicle hit Mr. Doe's car on the front passenger's side before coming to a halt. Complaining of pain with any movement of his neck, John was transported by ambulance to the emergency department of Wells Medical Center. X-rays of the cervical spine revealed an injury affecting his neck and back. He was placed on a high dose of anti-inflammatory medication and muscle relaxants and provided with a cervical collar. Because of the accident, John Doe has been unable to work since the motor vehicle accident in question.

Write the correct preposition in the blanks:

1. The study _____ diseases _____ the elderly is called geriatrics.

2. Proximal is _____ the point of attachment.

3. An oncologist is concerned _____ cancer.

4. Ventral and anterior pertain _____ the front of the body.

5. The patient lost much blood _____ the delivery of her child.

Supply a coordinating or correlative conjunction:

1. The responsibility belongs _____ to you _____ your assistant.

2. Make sure the patient is conscious enough to eat _____ swallow.

3. Explain the procedure _____ follow-up treatment.

4. _____ we obtain the blood test _____ we give glucose in the form of orange juice.

5. Each person may experience diabetes in his or her own unique way _____.

Write the corresponding part of speech from the list below above each italicized word in the sentences:

noun	**adverb**	**article**	**adjective**
pronoun	**preposition**	**conjunction**	**verb**

1. Patients facing death *pass* through many emotional and psychological stages.

2. Glucose tolerance testing is contraindicated for patients with recent surgery *or* myocardial infarctions.

3. *The* Patient's Bill of Rights is a set of laws that helps protect patients.

4. Occupational Safety and Health Administration, OSHA, suggests safety *measures* that must be taken to prevent or limit the spread of germs.

5. Limiting the use of antibiotics is crucial for the prevention of bacterial growth *and* resistance.

Answer the following questions:

1. Arrange these components as they would appear in a manuscript:

   References

   Appendix

   Abstract

   Results

Title page

Introduction

2. List four types of medical writings:

_____   _____

_____   _____

Select the word that describes the type of medical writing:

abstract	**report**	**writing style**
document	**manuscript**	**research**
appendix	**journal**	

1. Work submitted for publication. _____

2. Investigation into a topic to obtain facts or theories. _____

3. Short writing summarizing a larger work. _____

4. Item usually appearing in a newspaper or magazine. _____

5. Original writing that provides evidence or information. _____

Circle the correctly spelled word in each line:

1. Trendelanburg	Trendilenburg	Trendelenburg	Trendelonburg
2. hypirtension	hipertension	hypertision	hypertension
3. virus'	viruss	viruses	virusas
4. technikue	tehneque	tecknique	technique
5. urticaria	urtkaria	urtecaria	urtocaria
6. defencency	deficiency	dificiency	deficeincy
7. metaztazis	metatsasis	matastasis	metastasis
8. facia	fascia	faccsia	fassia
9. cianotic	cyantoic	cyanotic	ciaanotyc
10. diaphigm	diafragm	diaphragm	diephragm

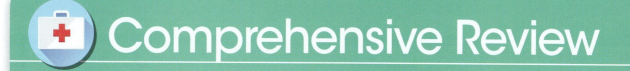

Comprehensive Review

Underline the Prepositional word(s) or phrase(s) that connect to other words in the sentence:

1. Before performing the procedure, wash your hands.
2. Investigation is a topic of facts and theories.
3. Common types of medical writings are documents and research papers.
4. Knowledge is listed among the qualities of a good doctor.
5. I'm calling because I cannot attend.
6. The doctor and lawyer came to a reasonable agreement.

Match the numbered words in Figure 8-6 with the words listed below:

article _____

noun _____

preposition _____

verb _____

adjective _____

predicate noun _____

conjunction _____

pronoun _____

adverb _____

prepositional phrase _____

direct object _____

complete subject _____

complete predicate _____

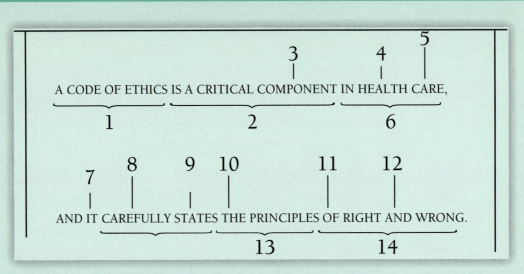

FIGURE 8-6 Dissecting a Sentence and Naming its Parts

MODULE 3

Putting It All Together

The Writing Process

Guidelines for Effective Writing

Objectives

After reading this section, the learner should be able to:

- implement the five stages of the writing process
- apply the criteria of a good writing style
- understand the advantages and disadvantages of writing on the computer
- spell various medical terms

Introduction

The most important word in the preceding subtitle is the word *process*. A process is a series of steps from beginning to end for achieving a desired result. Writing becomes easier when broken down into manageable steps. A process is not a one-step operation that magically produces a finished product on the first attempt. Many people wrongfully assume that once something is written, it is acceptable and the task is over. For both beginners and experienced writers, the implementation of all steps in the writing process is crucial to successful documentation. Dr. Seuss, a prestigious writer of children's literature, pondered hours and days on which preposition (to, of, for, by) conveyed the best meaning and rhythm.

In this section, the Writing Process Worksheet (see Appendix I) helps to facilitate the integration of this key process. The expectation is that learners will use this worksheet as they apply effective writing skills to medical reports, documents, and office correspondence. (Make copies of the Writing Process Worksheet so you can use it for the exercises in this chapter.)

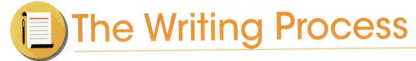

The Writing Process

The *writing process* includes five steps: prewriting, writing, rewriting, finalizing, and proofreading. These steps remain the same for any type of writing: a single sentence, narrative, speech, proposal, instruction, summary, description, paragraph, short story, novel, report, memo, or medical documentation. To demonstrate the steps of the writing process, we use a short paragraph on legal issues in health care as an example.

Step One: Prewriting

The *prewriting stage* is the planning stage, during which the author prepares an outline of everything he or she wants to write about the topic. At this initial step, the writer thinks about the reading audience and begins to focus more clearly on the subject. Details are jotted down in any order. If necessary, the author researches and limits the amount and length of writing. Correct spelling is not necessary at this stage. See Figure 9-1 for a sample of the prewriting process.

TOPIC	Legal Issues Affecting Health Care
SPECIFICS	Negligence
	Asault and batery
	Invasion of pivacy
NOTES	Research definitions
	Place issues in alphabetical order
	Have a good opening and closing sentence
	Keep the language simple
	Limit paragraph to five or six sentences

FIGURE 9-1 Prewriting Sample

Step Two: Writing

In the second step of the writing process is the *writing stage*, in which pencil is applied to paper or fingers to keyboard. The task is to start writing and keep it flowing. Forget about spelling, grammar, or punctuation at this point. Do not try to make things perfect. Just write. Let anything happen. Present facts or ideas about the topic. See Figure 9-2 for a sample of step two.

> The Patients bill of Rights require that patients be treated with respect Some violations against patients right are asault, negligence, invasion of privacy, verble abuse. Asault is verble or physical treats that cause harm, injury or fear. Failure to give proper care to patients is called negligense. Discussing information about patients publically without there soncent is unlawful. Failure to obey these areas make one lible or legally responsible.

FIGURE 9-2 Writing Sample

Step Three: Rewriting

In the *rewriting stage*, the manuscript is reviewed and refined. Read the first draft. Does it say what it is meant to say? Is the message clear and complete? Are facts or events in the right order? Does the writing follow the plan established in the prewriting stage? Concentrate on *each* word. Now correct grammar, spelling, and punctuation. (When using a computer, never depend solely on it to check spelling and grammar.) Change what needs to be changed. If necessary, consult others for feedback. Notice any satisfaction or discomfort that comes with reading the words. If there is discomfort, more work is needed. Review Figure 9-3 for the rewriting phase.

The Patients bill of Rights require that patients be treated with respect Some violations against patients rights are asault, negligence, invasion of privacy, verble abuse. Asault is verble or physical treats that cause harm, injury or fear. Failure to give proper care to patients is called negligense. Discussing information about patients publically without there soncent is unlawful. Failure to obey these areas make one lible or legally responsible.

FIGURE 9-3 Rewriting Sample

Note that proofreaders' marks can be used during the rewriting step. The most commonly used proofreaders' marks appear in Figure 9-4. In our age of technology, the paradigm is shifting away from

Symbol	Meaning	Symbol	Meaning
ds	double-space	—	insert underscore
ss	single-space	bold	boldface print
ital	use italic print	∧	insert a comma
⊙	insert a period	∨	insert an apostrophe
⁋	new paragraph	# ∧	insert space
⌣	delete a space; close up	⋏	insert a letter
sp	spell out	w/f	wrong font
∪	transpose		insert quotation marks
∧	insert a word	stet	let it stand
≡ or caps	capitalize	⌢	insert semicolon
ℓ	delete	⊙	insert colon
/ or lc	lowercase letter	⑦	insert question mark
=	insert a hyphen		

FIGURE 9-4 Proofreaders' Marks

writing on paper to typing on the computer. Proofreaders' marks are mentioned here for the traditional teachers and learners who may want to use them.

Step Four: Finalizing

Once all of the necessary corrections have been made to the writer's satisfaction, the final version is rewritten or retyped in the *finalizing stage*. Figure 9-5 shows the result of finalizing your work.

> The Patient's Bill of Rights requires that patients be treated with respect and dignity. Some violations against patient's rights are assault and battery, negligence, invasion of privacy, and verbal abuse. Assault and battery are verbal or physical treats that cause injury or fear. Failure to give proper care to patients is called negligence. Discussing information about patients without their consent is an invasion of privacy. Failure to obey these laws can have serious consequences.

FIGURE 9-5 Finalizing Sample

Step Five: Proofreading

The purpose of proofreading is to check and correct the final printed product. The *proofreading stage* is not the time to make major changes. It is the time to check for typing errors or slips of the pen. Mistakes reflect a negative image to the reader about the management of the medical office. Patients may assume or conclude that poor office performance means poor patient care. In the final copy of the sample paragraph resulting from step four (Figure 9-5), find the two errors that still remain.

In summary, it should be evident that good writing does not just happen. A writer must follow a systematic approach that calls for planning, organizing, writing, evaluating, and revising. Just as you learn to read by reading, you learn to write by writing. Writing improves with practice, and practice is the key to successful writing. When writing, it would be beneficial to use the five steps of the writing process. The Writing Process Worksheet and its thought processes are provided to help you with all your writing throughout your professional career.

 PRACTICE 1: The Writing Process

Using the five steps of the writing process, write a paragraph of approximately six to eight sentences on the topic of effective writing.

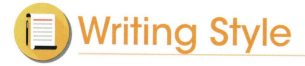

Writing Style

The dictionary defines the word *style* as a manner in which something is said, done, expressed, or performed. Style reveals how a writer thinks and feels about the people and situations that are the subjects of the writing. The two basic rules that apply to all types of writing are:

1. The writing style should be appropriate for the situation.
2. The writing style should be consistent throughout the writing.

Following are some of the criteria of a good writing style:

- *Purpose.* Initially, writers should know their audience and the purpose for which a particular writing task is being done. Is it to persuade, inform, entertain, or explain? Whatever the purpose, the writing must be clear, original, and focused on the message to be conveyed. What does the writer want the reader to understand? If the writer is not clear about the message, the reader will not be either. Writing is done for someone to read and should immediately engage the reader's interest.

  In a medical office setting, the purpose for writing is to document, transcribe, and organize patients' medical data in order to form a quality environment for good medical care.

> *No matter how technical a subject, all writing is done for human beings by human beings.*
>
> Jacqueline Berke

- *Appropriate Wording.* Writing style is developed from a series of choices that makes the writer's style unique. One of those choices involves the words that are used. Words are combined to convey an intended meaning or attitude. A message with the same meaning can be written in many different ways for different situations.

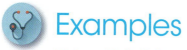 # Examples

His heart is fluttering.

His heart flutters whenever he sees you.

His heart is in tachycardia.

The patient has tachycardia.

The rate of heart palpitations has reached a serious level.

This medicine does things to my heart.

The patient has an increased heart rate.

My heart is all worked up over this health problem.

The style of writing for a newspaper is quite different from that of a novel, textbook, romance, research paper, biography, poem, narrative, short story, business letter, autobiography, or medical report. The writing style of the medical profession is unique. In medical documentation, writing is brief and detailed.

To be skilled in the style of medical documentation, knowledge of medical terms is of utmost importance. Use words that are precise and concise so the reader can easily understand what is said.

> *Doctors bury their mistakes. Lawyers hang them. Journalists put their mistakes on the front page.*
>
> Anonymous

- *Explicitness.* Good writing avoids generalization and is as specific as possible.

General	Patient says he has pain in the back.
Specific	Pt. states he has low back pain in the lumbar region.
General	The patient suffered from pain.
Specific	The patient suffered from a migraine headache.
General	The physician began the treatment.
Specific	The physician reluctantly began the treatment.
General	The patient is coughing after surgery.
Specific	Patient is coughing/deep breathing every 15 min. while awake.

> *Trim sentences, like trim bodies, usually require far more effort than flabby ones.*
>
> Clair Kehrwald Cook

- *Conciseness.* A complete message stated in as few words as possible and without unnecessary words is another feature of good writing style.

Wordy	The patient was violent, abusive, and was hitting the nurse.
Clearer	Patient showed violent behavior.
Wordy	Place the reports in the file. After the reports are in the file, put them in alphabetical order.
Clearer	File the reports alphabetically.
Wordy	The reason I was late was due to the fact that my alarm clock didn't ring.
Clearer	I was late because I forgot to set the alarm.

> *The beautiful part of writing is that you don't have to get it right the first time, unlike, say, a brain surgeon.*
>
> Robert Cormier

- *Correct Grammar.* The use of good grammar is usually equated with writing well. Although the two are interconnected, one does not necessarily guarantee the other. While it may be useful to learn isolated skills at times, grammatical concepts must be learned by integrating them into the context of writing. Writers must transfer what they learn from studying grammar to their own writing.
- *Smoothness.* The use of transitional words to unite one sentence or paragraph with another helps to eliminate bumps or rough spots. Each sentence or paragraph should lead clearly and logically to the next, providing a smooth flow of ideas.

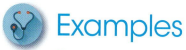 # Examples

The x-rays were negative. *Therefore,* additional testing is unnecessary.

The patient didn't follow directions when using the medication. *Consequently,* her blood pressure reading was invalid.

- *Inclusive Language.* All types of medical writing should contain gender-free language. At one point in history, nursing was considered only a woman's career and most physicians were men:

  The doctor and his patients . . . The nurse and her patients . . .

The use of the word *his* often implies both men and women.

  The hospital employee must sign *his* name.

Some feel that one way to overcome non-inclusive language is to use both *his* and *her* together.

  The hospital employee signed *his/her* name.

Many professionals feel that the *his/her* combination is awkward. Two ways to avoid its use are (1) by changing nouns to their plural form and using the pronoun *their,* and (2) by rewriting the sentence to avoid using a pronoun.

  Hospital employees must sign *their* benefit plans.

  All hospital employees must sign benefit plans.

Use of gender-free language in written (and spoken) language fosters equality in the workplace. Note how gender-specific terms have changed over the years.

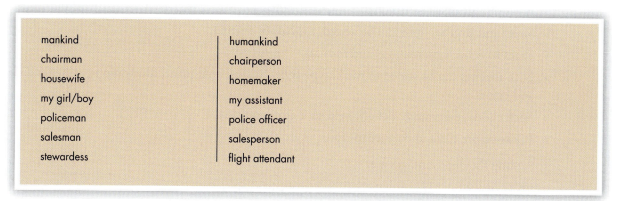

mankind	humankind
chairman	chairperson
housewife	homemaker
my girl/boy	my assistant
policeman	police officer
salesman	salesperson
stewardess	flight attendant

Developing a good writing style requires commitment to the writing process. Writing is hard work and needs constant editing and revising. No matter how experienced a writer, there is always room for improvement. The health care professional must be committed to the writing process in order to give the task the proper attention it needs and the practice it requires. Practice is the key to becoming a good writer. Practice is what makes good writing better. All writings possess the challenge to improve. Good writing is achieved by working and reworking ideas again and again.

Finally, learning to write well goes beyond good grammar skills, proofreading, revising, and organizing. Developing writing skills also comes from reading the works of good writers.

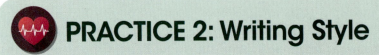

PRACTICE 2: Writing Style

Rewrite to simplify these sentences:

1. I can't tell you, Doctor, how I really, really appreciate what you did for me. _____

2. Working in the operating room, the nurse did not see the doctor. _____

3. Cathy was Dr. Villmare's medical assistant. She worked two years for him. _____

4. Read the medical report literally, word for word. _____

5. It is the hospital's intention to issue bonuses based on a worker's performance. _____

Computer Writing

The computer is an assistant in the writing process. A computer is a writer's best friend, if the writer has keyboard, writing, and computer skills. If the student is competent in two of these skills, the other skill can be learned. Otherwise, using the computer to improve writing may be counterproductive.

The advantages to using a computer far outweigh the disadvantages for many reasons:

- The computer is faster than longhand writing.
- The writer can focus more freely on ideas.
- The writer can endure longer periods of writing time and cover a topic more thoroughly.
- Revisions are easier to make.
- Small and large sections can be added, moved, or deleted.
- Pages have uniform margins and formats.
- Nice touches can be added to work: type styles, italics, bold print, illustrations, tables and charts, and colors.
- Spell check and grammar check help spot errors quickly.
- Printouts are clean and easier to read.

Among the disadvantages are:

- The writer has to continually stop and read what was written.
- Some errors, such as missing words, commas, and periods, are hard to see on the screen.
- For some writers, revising, rereading, and evaluating from the screen are more difficult than from a paper.
- The writer must remember to SAVE the material. Not all software has an automatic SAVE feature.

Guidelines for Effective Writing Summary

The Writing Process:	A series of steps for achieving effective writing.
1. Prewriting	Outline the topics to include in the writing.
2. Writing	Write and keep it flowing, without regard to correct spelling, grammar, or punctuation.
3. Rewriting	Correct errors and determine if the message is clear.
4. Finalizing	Write or type the final copy.
5. Proofreading	Check the final version for remaining errors.

Characteristics of Good Writing	
Purpose	Understand why a message is written.
Appropriate wording	Use the style that fits the message.
Explicitness	Avoid generalizations and be specific.
Conciseness	State the message once and in as few words as possible.
Correct grammar	Transfer grammar skills to writing.
Smoothness	Use transitional words to unite sentences.
Inclusive language	Use gender-free language.

Medical Spelling

Become familiar with the spelling of the following words:

absorbent	diarrhea	necessary	reiterated
accessible	eligible	occurrence	rheumatism
accommodation	flatulence	opportunity	severity
analysis	hemorrhage	palliative	successful
analyze	hygiene	perseverance	sufficient
beneficial	inadvertently	precede	susceptible
canceled	infectious	prescription	suture
conscious	intermittent	procedure	tachycardia
comparative	irritated	quantity	technique
convalescent	irrigated	recurrence	umbilicus
deficiency	judgment	referral	xiphoid

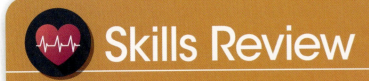

Skills Review

Answer true or false to the following statements:

1. A writer with good grammar skills will automatically write well. _____

2. Reading the works of famous authors can help improve one's writing. _____

3. Ordinarily the works of good experienced writers don't need much revision. _____

4. The purpose of a topic sentence is to tie ideas together. _____

5. For an experienced writer, skipping a stage of the writing process is allowed. _____

6. Writing for health care personnel consists mainly of transcribing medical manuscripts. _____

7. Correct spelling and grammar are necessary through all phases of the writing process. _____

8. If one word conveys a clear message, use it. _____

9. A broad vocabulary makes reading more interesting. _____

10. The informal writing style for medical personnel should exclude abbreviations. _____

Circle the letter of the best-constructed sentence in each group:

1. A. Because patients pay the bill, invoices are their responsibility.

   B. Invoices are the patients' responsibility.

   C. Medical assistants send invoices to patients.

2. A. When the patient was young, the patient had frequent urinary tract infections as a child.

   B. The patient had urinary tract infections as a child.

   C. The patient had frequent urinary tract infections as a child.

3. A. Most likely, the syndrome is viral hepatitis.

  B. I thought the syndrome presented viral hepatitis.

  C. The syndrome is thought by me to be most likely viral hepatitis.

4. A. I am thrilled that you referred this pleasant, beautiful patient to me.

  B. Thank you for referring this patient for neurological evaluation.

  C. Thank you for the reference.

5. A. Avoidance of the infection is the best approach.

  B. Avoidance of the infection includes polio vaccination.

  C. Avoidance includes vaccination of anyone with the disease.

Use the Writing Process Worksheet to complete.

Explain why you want to be a medical professional.

Circle the correctly spelled word in each line:

1. perservirance	perseverance	preseverance	preseverence
2. paliative	palliative	paleative	palleative
3. necsesary	nessessary	necessary	necissary
4. prescription	perscripition	perscription	prescishun
5. rhumatism	ruematism	rhuematism	rheumatism
6. acomodation	accomodation	accommodation	acommodation
7. benificial	beneficial	benefecial	beneficle
8. ocurrence	occurence	occurrance	occurrence
9. intermittent	intermrmittant	intermittant	intermitant
10. diarhea	diarea	diarrhhea	diarrhea

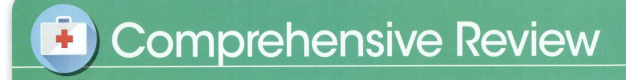
Comprehensive Review

Use the Writing Process Worksheet to summarize this paragraph in your own words.

Hand washing is one important step that helps limit the spread of germs. Before and after contact with each patient, wet your hands and wrists. Work soap into lather, getting between fingers and under nails. Lower hands with fingernails downward and rinse well. Dry your hands carefully with a paper towel. Turn off the water tap with a paper towel to avoid any germs on the faucet. Apply lotion if desired.

The Writing Process Worksheet

1. PREWRITING – write down facts, organize ideas

   _____   _____

   _____   _____

   _____   _____

   _____   _____

   _____   _____

2. WRITING – write without concern for grammar or punctuation

   _____

   _____

   _____

   _____

   _____

   _____

   _____

3. REWRITING – correct grammar, make changes using proofreaders' marks

   _____

   _____

   _____

   _____

   _____

_____

_____

4. FINALIZING – type or write final copy

_____

_____

_____

_____

_____

5. PROOFREAD – read the final copy aloud for a final check

_____

_____

_____

_____

_____

SECTION 10
The Resume and Cover Letter

Objectives

After reading this section, the learner should be able to:

- write a resume
- use appropriate words in the resume
- write a cover letter

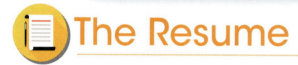

The Resume

The *resume* is an account of your skills, progress, and career highlights. It takes energy and thought. Over 500 years ago it was an introductory letter. It is now a very important reference for employers when interviewing a prospective employee.

Essentials of the Resume

List on a sheet of paper these essential pieces of information. Think in the Writing Process mode.

- Contact information: You need to list your contact information. Your address, email, and preferably your cell phone are necessary parts of your resume. It is the way the employer will contact you for an interview and ultimately for your new job.

- Related skills: List your skills and any pertinent related experiences. Keep in mind your new employer wants to know that you have the ability to handle the job. You are marketing your ability to listen and learn. You are marketing your ability to "get things done." Be selective and impressive.

- Education: You may want to include your education. Listing the school and some of the courses. Some of your courses may be very relevant and important to the employer, especially if you are just out of school. Do list your honors or accomplishments.
- Certifications: You may want to list your certification. Are you certified through the *American Association of Medical Assistants (AAMA)* as a Certified Medical Assistant (CMA)?
- Memberships/conferences: If you should have membership in any professional organizations such as the AAMA. Have you gone to any local conferences? Meetings? Are you involved in the professional organizations?
- References: Employers like references. You will be asked to list references at some point. Many employers want to check and be sure you are reliable and you actually have the talent for the job. Always contact your references first to notify them that they may be called. Many times the employer will ask for letters of recommendation. These should be included with your resume.

Your Objective

The objective usually comes right after your contact information. It is important to choose an objective, job objective, work objective, career objective, or career goal. Keep this statement short. It tells the employer what you want to do. This may be the hardest, but it is selling your skills. It tells your employer what you want. It will show the employer you are the candidate for this job. Keep it clear and focused. This is the first statement the new employer reads. The objective and the current job opportunities should match. You do not want to be mentioning your objective to be "a clinical assistant" when your past jobs have been in retail. It is best not to mention the retail jobs.

The objective may be the reason the employer calls you for the interview. Be as specific as possible. There is another theory that the objective may be mentioned in the cover letter rather than the resume. The reasoning is that the employer may not consider you if the resume objective is too specific or too general. Stating it in a letter may help you explain the objective better.

The Importance of Keywords

Employers may put resumes that are emailed on a searchable data base. Even if the resume is mailed it may be put on a scanner, converted to a file, and loaded onto a large computer database. It is an applicant tracking system, often referred to as ATS. It is a recruitment tool for employers. The database is growing in popularity as the search for jobs grow. The ATS or character recognition scans the resumes to find certain words. It searches keywords that match skills, schools, years of experiences, certifications, awards, and job titles.

It is important to know if you are emailing a resume or going through snail mail. Electronic software may filter the application automatically. Many keywords will bring your resume through the software search. Here are some points that will help the download of your resume:

- Remove tabs and indents.
- Remove italics, underlines, bold, and graphics.
- Remove horizontal and vertical lines.
- Use asterisks to highlight achievements, rather than bullets.
- Save the file in basic Courier, Calibri, or a similar font.

When writing your resume, you should use action words.

Powerful Action Words

administered	assigned	authorized	controlled
supervised	addressed	arranged	collaborated
communicated	reported	responded	initiated
summarized	computed	constructed	instituted
programmed	specialized	studied	increased
utilized	executed	improved	led
corresponded	discussed	explained	influenced
analyzed	conducted	determined	explored
detected	diagnosed	evaluated	examined
identified	gathered	interpreted	interviewed
formulated	adapted	coordinated	researched
clarified	coached	advised	conducted
contributed	transformed	succeeded	surpassed
improved	facilitated	informed	systematized
observed	negotiated	marketed	participated
trained	assessed	guided	provided
rehabilitated	presented	scheduled	submitted
recorded	processed	encouraged	educated
demonstrated	transformed	spearheaded	pioneered
exceeded	created	retrieved	adapted
creative skills	cataloged	cared for	distributed

Types of Resumes

There are three basic types of resumes:

1. chronological
2. functional
3. hybrid/combination

The *chronological resume* lists your career/work history in a traditional format from the most recent to the earliest (reverse chronological order). It is usually done by listing the dates. The most recent job is posted first with your skills. It can be done with bullet points. Employers like to look and easily see where and what jobs you have held. People who have a very strong consistent work history would benefit from this resume. Figure 10-1 shows a sample of a chronological resume.

The *functional resume* is a focus on skills first. It is about the important skills you have been using. It describes your activities and accomplishments using the skills. The details of your skills come first and your employment history is secondary. Use this if you are in the middle of a transition or career change.

Name

Address

Email and phone number

Job Objective: The reason you want the job (be specific)

Summary of Work Experience:

20XX–20XX   Work Title, City, State

                   Skills used. Experience. Positive action words

19XX–20XX   Work Title, City, State

                   Any problems solved

                   Accomplishments

19XX–19XX   Work Title, City, State

                   Volunteer

                   Awards. Use those positive action verbs

Education:

19XX–19XX   Degree, major

                   University

                   Post High school career school

                   Certifications

FIGURE 10-1 Sample Chronological Resume

Use this if there is a gap in your employment history. Very often recent graduates will use this form. Figure 10-2 shows a sample of a functional resume.

The *hybrid/combination resume* gives details about the skills and experiences within the chronological work history. Sometimes this is used with an imperfect work history. Perhaps your work history is spotty and you wish to change your career path. This is often tailored to the specific job. Use this if you are applying for a certain type of employment. Figure 10-3 shows an example of a hybrid resume.

Name

Address

Email and Phone

Job Objective: Positive specific words/your reason for wanting this job.

Education and Skills/Qualifications:

Career school, College, Degree, GPA, Dean's list, Major, Concentration

Courses:

Specific to this job

Skills that relate to your new career and profession.

Positive action verbs that pertain to the career job you are applying for:

Work History: (if applicable)

20XX–20XX   Work Title, City, State

              Skills used. Powerful verbs that might relate to your transitioned career change.

FIGURE 10-2 Sample Functional Resume

Wrapping It Up

Decide the type of resume you would like to use. Write and rewrite … proofread and proofread again.

Let it rest. Go back to the resume at a later time and reread and ask yourself if this is what you would like … if you were the employer.

Try to keep the resume to one page. However, two pages are okay if it means including important skills. Note that employers don't like looking at two page resumes. They tend to be long and contain useless information about hobbies and personal likes and dislikes. One page is usually best.

The typeface should be easy to read. The size should be between 10 and 12 points. Please don't hyphenate words or violate the margins. Margins are usually 1 inch all around. If needed, margins can be shortened to .75 inch or widened to 1.5 inches. Create a neat looking resume.

It is best to use white, off white, or ivory paper. Bonded paper always gives a better impression. It tells the human resource person or the employer that you took time and care in your presentation of yourself.

Name

Address

Email and Phone

Career Objective: Very specific to this job you are applying for.

Profile:

    List your achievements, awards, and skills that pertain to this job specifically.

    What specific clinical skills did you learn and use?

    What administrative courses are relevant?

    Did you excel in any particular area?

    What was your professional experience?

    Use the keywords that are powerful and positive.

    Certifications.

Education and Certification:

20XX   Certified

Affiliations: If applicable

Employment History:

20XX–20XX   If this is applicable.

FIGURE 10-3 Sample Hybrid Resume

The Cover Letter

The cover letter increases the chance that the prospective, potential employer will look at your resume, interview you, and eventually hire you. The cover letter is the captivating vehicle that decides whether the new employer will either look at your resume for an interview or throw it in the rejection basket. It is important the cover letter captures the reader's attention.

Because of the Internet, applying for a job has changed drastically from 15 years ago. Resumes are often emailed or faxed. One of the best ways to grab the attention of the employer is to write a clean, concise, incredible, eye catching cover letter.

The cover letter often conveys your personality and your efficiency. If it is sloppy, it will relay inefficiency. If it is poorly keyed or typed with errors, it will lead to the rejection basket. Deliver an impact.

Convey enthusiasm and a positive attitude. Keep the cover letter to one page, short and sweet. The people reading your letter probably have many other letters to read, so capture their attention with your skills and ability to convey that you are the right person for the job. Above all, let your letter show confidence that you are capable and can handle the job extremely well. Always include your contact information. Figure 10-4 shows a sample cover letter.

Your Return address

Typed here along with

Your Email and phone

Date here, 20XX

Name and

Address to whom

You are sending the cover letter

Dear XXXX:

It is with great interest that I send you my resume applying for the position advertised in the Florida Sunday Daily News. I am optimistic that my qualifications will complement the job.

Enclosed is my resume for the position of _____, as published in the Florida (be specific) newspaper. I feel very confident that my skills meet your expectations.

I am currently graduating from _____. My experience in the clinical and administrative courses gave me a wonderful learning opportunity. I have taken ECGs, medical histories, blood work, and performed many other clinical and administrative tasks.

I look forward to meeting with you for an interview at any time during the week. Thank you so much for your time in this matter. You may contact me at (555) 555-5555.

Sincerely,

(Your Signature)

Your Name

Enclosure, Resume

FIGURE 10-4 Sample Cover Letter

Skills Review

True or False

1. Contact information is not needed on your resume, only in your cover letter. _____

2. The objective should be clear, concise, and relative to the job. _____

3. References are always needed at the end of the resume. _____

4. A cover letter says thank you for the interview. _____

5. A resume is needed only if you see an ad in the newspaper. _____

6. A resume is your opportunity to promote your special skills. _____

7. Powerful words produce a high impact. _____

8. A resume is about your life. _____

9. Proofreading is essential when sending a resume to a potential employer. _____

10. The resume is the single most important job search document. _____

Comprehensive Review

Write your practice resume:

1. Use three of your most important skills that you have learned in your program.

2. Keep your resume to one page.

3. Concentrate on using powerful, high-impact keywords.

4. Be honest.

Write your practice cover letter:

1. Include your contact information.

2. Be positive.

3. Write an encouraging statement that you would love to meet for an interview with your prospective employer.

Appendix A:
Spelling Rules

Spelling correctly is a real challenge. Many medical terms are long, uncommon, and somewhat tricky: *tourniquet, pneumonia, scirrhous, diarrhea, ecchymosis,* and *herniorrhaphy.* The allied health professional must be careful about spelling, especially since medical reports are legal documents. Sometimes the incorrect use of simple words like *their* and *there* or *its* and *it's* is easily overlooked by the careful eye of the most conscientious proofreader. (In the word *conscientious,* does the *i* come before the *e* or the *e* before the *i*?)

When uncertain about how to spell a word, it should become a habit to look it up in the dictionary. A good idea for allied health workers is to keep an ongoing list of words that are most often misspelled in a small pocket notebook. Such lists of misspelled words differ from person to person, but the effort of compiling these lists can be rewarding.

Another helpful hint in building spelling efficiency is to divide words and spell them syllable by syllable. However, words are often misspelled because they are not pronounced correctly. In many words, letters are silent. One example is the word *often.* According to the dictionary, the first pronunciation of the word *often* sounds like *offen.* Spelling the word as it sounds is often incorrect.

Knowledge of a few basic spelling rules is helpful when documenting medical reports. Following are rules applicable in four basic areas that make spelling easier.

1. **Using *ei* or *ie***
   - In most words, the letter *i* goes before *e: chief, view, piece, quiet, brief, hygiene, achieve, relief, grief, believe, review, friend, orient, belief,* and *died.*
   - The letter *i* goes before *e* after the *sh* sound: *shield, patient, proficient,* and *species.*
   - When the letters *i* and *e* are sounded separately, the spelling is easier: *sci-ence, a-li-en,* and *ex-pe-ri-ence.*
   - The letter *i* goes before *e* except after the letter *c: receipt, receive, conceive, ceiling, perceive, deceive,* and *conceit.* Exceptions include *leisure, height, weird, seize, foreign, Alzheimers, neither,* and *either.*
   - The letter *e* goes before *i* when *ei* sounds like the letter *a: weigh, weight, neighbor, their, heir, reign, veil,* and *eight.*
   - Change *ie* to *y* before adding *ing: die = dying, lie = lying.*

2. Doubling the Final Consonant

A student wrote about an experience that she had when trying to secure gainful employment as a medical assistant:

I recently graduated from a medical assistant course and hopped to secure a position in a medical office. During one interview, I was given many pre-programed tests to determine if I possesed the potential to handle the job. I was quized on the many tasks required of a medical assistant. Initially I reactted calmly to the test. It never oc-cured to me that I would find anything difficult. One of the exercises was to proofread a document written by a doctor who transfered a patient from one hospital to another. Because the physician refered the patient to another specialist, there was a lot of information. I regreted only that the test took so long to complete. After two weeks, I was notiffied that someone else received the position. I wondered why.

The most predominant spelling error in this paragraph involves whether to double or not double the final consonant. The final consonant is doubled when the following criteria are met:

- The word is one syllable: *fit.*
- The word ends in a single consonant: *fit.*
- The final consonant is preceded by a vowel or the letter y: fit.
- What is added (the suffix) begins with a vowel: *ed* or *ing.*

Under these conditions, the final consonant is doubled: *fitted.* Here are other examples:

ship + ed = shipped	run + ing = running
hot + est = hottest	ship + ing = shipping

Exceptions to this rule involve words ending in the letter *w (showing)* or *x (boxed),* and the word *bus.*

What happens to words of more than one syllable? Double the final consonant in words of more than one syllable under these conditions:

- The accent must be on the last syllable: re*gret.*
- The ending must be a single consonant: regre*t.*
- The last letter is preceded by one vowel: regr*e*t.
- What is added begins with a vowel: *ed* or *ing.*

When all these conditions are present, double the final consonant: *regretted.* Here are other examples:

transfer + ed = transferred	transfer + ing = transferring
occur + ed = occurred	occur + ence = occurrence
acquit + ed = acquitted	acquit + ing = acquitting

A critical point to remember about this rule is that a dictionary is necessary to be sure that the accent is on the last syllable of the word.

Another way to look at this rule is to identify when NOT to double the final consonant:

- When the accent is *not* on the last syllable: *offer, offering.*
- The word does *not* end in a single consonant: *cold, colder.*
- The last letter is *not* preceded by a *single* vowel: ob*tain, obtained.*
- What is added does *not* begin with a vowel: *ness,* goodness.

Examples

differ + ent = *different,* the accent is not on the last syllable.

cancel + ed = *canceled,* the accent is on the first syllable.

leap + ed = *leaped,* there are two vowels before the final consonant.

film + ed = *filmed,* the word ends in two consonants instead of one.

There are, of course, exceptions. Many words in the dictionary have two acceptable spellings.

Examples

travel + ers = *travelers* or *travellers*

counsel + or = *counselor* or *counsellor*

label + ed = *labeled* or *labelled*

program + ing = *programming* or *programing*

3. **Adding Suffixes to a Final Silent *e***

What happens to the letter *e* at the end of a word when a suffix is added, particularly when the *e* is silent? Several rules help to answer that question.

- Drop the final *e* before adding a suffix that begins with a vowel:

Examples:	Exceptions:
state + ing = *stating*	eye + ing = *eyeing*
like + ing = *liking*	dye + ing = *dyeing*
use + ing = *using*	shoe + ing = *shoeing*

- Do not drop the final *e* if the suffix begins with a consonant:

Examples:	Exceptions:
state + ment = *statement*	judge + ment = judgment
like + ness = *likeness*	acknowledge + ment = acknowledgment
use + ful = *useful*	
awe + some = *awesome*	

- Do not drop the *e* from words ending in *ce* or *ge* when adding *able* or *ous:*

notice + able = *noticeable*

outrage + ous = *outrageous*

- Drop the *e* before adding the suffix *y:*

edge + y = *edgy*

ice + y = *icy*

- When the word ends in *ie* and the suffix begins with *i,* change the *i* to *y* and add the suffix:

vie + ing = vying

untie + ing = untying

4. Adding Suffixes to Words Ending in *y* and *c*

- For words ending in *y* preceded by a consonant, change the *y* to *i* before adding a suffix:

Examples: Exception:

fancy + ful = fanc*i*ful   shy + ness = *shyness*

glory + ous = glor*i*ous

accompany + ment = accompan*i*ment

happy + ness = happ*i*ness

- For words ending in *y* preceded by a vowel, keep the *y* before adding the suffix:

annoy + ance = annoyance
obey + ed = obeyed

Although these four basic rules seem lengthy, common sense dictates their usage. They concretize and reinforce spelling habits writers already practice.

Appendix B:
Capitalization Rules

Capitalize the following except as noted:

Rules:	**Examples:**
The pronoun *I*	After *I* read the book, you can have it.
The first word in a sentence	*P*oems are made by fools like me.
People's names	*R*oberta, *F. S*cott *F*itzgerald
Titles as part of a person's name	*S*enator *K*ennedy, *P*rime *M*inister *A*bouti
Do *not* capitalize a title used without a person's name.	secretary of state, the senator from Ohio
Words like mother, father, aunt, uncle used alone.	I asked *M*other to go.
Do *not* capitalize family members when accompanied by a possessive pronoun.	I asked my *m*other to go.
Title after a name	Jonathan Harlan, *M.D.*, Randy Kane, *Jr.*
Geographic names, streets, towns, and regions of a country.	*C*hina, *D*ade *C*ounty, *W*est *S*ide, the *S*outheast, *R*odeo *D*rive, *F*rance, *A*tlantic *O*cean
Do *not* capitalize directions.	Drive *w*est. Face *s*outh.
Languages, races.	*S*panish, *F*rench accent, *B*lack history
Do *not* capitalize *the* before these names.	*t*he Nile River, *t*he French people
Important buildings or structures	*V*ietnam *M*emorial, *T*rump *T*ower
Historical ages, events	*R*omantic *E*ra, *S*enior *P*rom
Do *not* capitalize *the* before these names.	*t*he Senior Prom
Names of products	*A*von, *B*ayer
Names of companies, stores, banks	*D*elta *A*irlines, *M*ercy *M*edical *C*enter, *P*athology *D*epartment, *F*ord truck

Names of specific courses	*English Grammar 101*
Do *not* capitalize subject matter.	*English grammar*
Organizations	*American Medical Association, Special Olympics*
Political parties	*Democrat, Republican*
Religions, deities, worshipped figures	*Baptist, Judaism, Catholicism, Buddha, Christ, Allah, God, Bible, Promised Land*
Important words in the title of a book, movie, etc.	*Bill of Rights, Gray's Anatomy*
Unless they are the first word in a title, articles and prepositions are *not* capitalized.	*The Grapes of Wrath, The Return of the Native*
Holidays, days of the week, months	*Christmas, Sunday, July, Hanukkah*
Do *not* capitalize seasons.	*spring, summer, winter, fall*
Do *not* capitalize academic years.	*freshman, sophomore, junior, senior*
First word in a direct quote	*"The pain is here," said Mary.* *Mary said, "The pain is here."*
Do *not* capitalize the first word of the continuation of an interrupted quote.	*"The pain," said Mary, "is in the stomach."*
Eponyms	*Parkinson's disease, Babinski's reflex, Apgar score, Fowler's position, Bell's palsy, Epstein-Barr virus*
Certain abbreviations	B.C. Ph.D. A.D. M.D.

Appendix C:
Number Use

- In general, spell out numbers ten and under: one, four, six, nine.
- Use figures for numbers over ten: 16, 26, 785, 591.
- Spell out numbers used as the first word in a sentence: Sixteen x-rays were taken.
- Spell out indefinite numbers and amounts: a few hundred dollars, a bunch of fifties.
- Be consistent with numbers in a sentence: five computers and twelve scanners; 5 computers, 16 scanners, and 24 laptops.
- When two numbers modify the same noun, spell out one (the shorter number) and use numerals for the other: We mailed over 200 five-page reports.
- Separate unrelated numbers with a comma: On July 1, 28 people were laid off from work.
- A fraction alone is written in words with a hyphen: Three-fourths of the population go to bed hungry.
- Use numerals for mixed fractions: Give her 1½ ounces of medicine.
- Use figures with a.m., p.m.: 11:30 a.m., 6:15 p.m.

  Note: Omit :00 on the hour time: 7 a.m.
  Do not use a.m. and p.m. with the word *o'clock:* The meeting is at 4 o'clock.
- Always use figures with symbols and abbreviations: pH 7.5, 33%, # 21 gauge, 2 cc. t.i.d., 3+, pulses 2+.
- Use figures with drugs: Give 75 milligrams of Meperidine Intramuscular.
- When the day precedes the month, use ordinal endings (-th, -rd, -nd, -st): The 2nd of February is my anniversary.
- Spell out an ordinal with no month: It is my twenty-eighth wedding anniversary.
- Spell out street names under 10: Fifth Avenue.
- Use numerals for all house numbers but one: She lives at One 24th Street.
- Use numerals for money: 45 cents, $3.45, $15 for membership.

Notes: Use the word *cents* for amounts under a dollar. Use a dollar sign for money over one dollar. Omit .00 with even dollars.

- Use numerals for ages: The patient is 46 yrs. old. John is 16 years and 2 months old.
- Use numerals with numbers that have decimal fractions: An incision was made 4.5 cm below. . . .

   Note: Always put a zero before a decimal that is not a whole number: Two capsules of Marcaine 0.2% were used.

- Dimensions, sizes, and temperature readings are expressed in figures: 43° below zero; My shoe size is 6½, and I weigh 120 lbs.

Arabic and Roman Numerals

1	I	20	XX
2	II	30	XXX
3	III	40	XL
4	IV	50	L
5	V	60	LX
6	VI	70	LXX
7	VII	80	LXXX
8	VIII	90	XC
9	IX	100	C
10	X	200	CC
11	XI	300	CCC
12	XII	400	CD
13	XIII	500	D
14	XIV	600	DC
15	XV	700	DCC
16	XVI	800	DCCC
17	XVII	900	CM
18	XVIII	1000	M
19	XIX		

Appendix D:
Clichés

A cliché is a word or phrase that has lost its effectiveness through overuse. There are thousands of clichés in the English language. Following are some examples:

after all is said and done	food for thought
as luck would have it	fresh as a daisy
as old as the hills	golden opportunity
at a later date	good as my word
better late than never	grin and bear it
busy as a bee	in a nutshell
by leaps and bounds	in one ear and out the other
calm before the storm	in the final analysis
cart before the horse	in the nick of time
cool as a cucumber	it goes without saying
crystal clear, clear as a bell	knowing the ropes
days are numbered	lap of luxury
dead as a doornail	last but not least
don't rock the boat	lesser of two evils
easier said than done	light as a feather
few and far between	miss the boat
finger in every pie	more than meets the eye
fish out of water	no time like the present
flat as a pancake	playing with fire
fly off the handle	put your foot in your mouth
quick as a wink	sink or swim
raining cats and dogs	skating on thin ice

red as a beet

regular as clockwork

safe and sound

see eye to eye

short and sweet

shot in the arm

snug as a bug in a rug

so far so good

straight as an arrow

tough as nails

without rhyme or reason

Because clarity and conciseness are so essential in medical documentation, clichés should not be used. Notice how clichés in this memo distort its meaning:

Re: Stress Management Workshop

Believe it or not, Williams Hospital is offering a workshop on Stress Management. The cost of the workshop is a drop in the bucket compared to the benefits received. Applicants will come through with flying colors and learn how to be good to themselves. First and foremost, they will learn how to relate to difficult people, save time, and handle stress. This is just the icing on the cake. If you should feel that you are not satisfied, your costs will be returned. Leave no stone unturned. Openings are few and far between. Put your best foot forward and apply today.

Appendix E:
Titles and Salutations

Effective letters require that the appropriate titles and salutations be used.

Position or Title	Styling for Address	Styling for Salutation
Executive branch of the federal government		
the president	The Honorable (full name) President of the United States The White House	Dear Mr. President:
wife of president	Mrs. (full name) The White House	Dear Mrs. (surname):
vice president	The Honorable (full name) Vice President of the United States	Dear Mr. Vice President:
cabinet member	The Honorable (full name) Secretary of _____ The Secretary of _____	Dear Mr. Secretary:
attorney general	The Honorable (full name) The Attorney General	Dear Mr. Attorney General:
postmaster general	The Honorable (full name) The Postmaster General	Dear Mr. Postmaster General:
commissioner	The Honorable (full name) Commissioner of _____	Dear Mr. Commissioner: Dear Madam Commissioner: Dear Mr. (full name): Dear Ms. (full name):
chief justice	The Honorable (full name) The Chief Justice of the United States	Dear Mr. (Madam) Chief Justice:
federal judge	The Honorable (full name) Judge of _____	Dear Judge (surname):

director or head of an agency	The Honorable (full name) (title, name of agency)	Dear Mr./Mrs./Ms. (surname):

Members of congress

senator	The Honorable (full name) United States Senate	Dear Senator (surname):
Representative	The Honorable (full name) House of Representatives	Dear Representative (surname):
Speaker of the House	The Honorable (full name) Speaker of the House of Representatives	Dear Mr. Speaker: Dear Madam Speaker:
Chairman of a Committee	The Honorable (full name) Chairman of _____	Dear Mr. Chairman: Dear Madam Chairman:
Librarian of Congress	The Honorable (full name) Librarian of Congress	Dear Mr./Mrs./Ms.(surname):

American diplomatic officials

Ambassador	The Honorable (full name) American Ambassador	Dear Mr./Madam Ambassador:
Minister	The Honorable (full name) American Minister	Dear Mr./Madam Minister:
Chargé d'Affaires	(full name), Esq. American Chargé d'Affaires	Dear Mr./Madam Chargé d'Affaires:
Consul	(full name), Esq. American Consul	Dear Mr./Mrs./Ms.(surname):
Representative to the United Nations	The Honorable (full name) United States Representative to the United Nations	Dear Mr./Mrs./Ms.(surname):

Foreign diplomatic officials

Foreign Ambassador	His/Her Excellency (full name)	Dear Mr./Madam Ambassador:
British Ambassador	His/Her Excellency The Right Honorable (full name)	Dear Mr./Madam Ambassador:
Chargé d'Affaires	Mr./Mrs./Ms. (full name) Chargé d'Affaires of _____	Dear Mr./Madam Chargé d'Affaires:
Consul	The Honorable (full name) Consul of _____	Dear Sir/Madam:
Minister	The Honorable (full name) Minister of _____	Dear Mr./Madam Minister:
Prime Minister	His/Her Excellency (full name)	Excellency Dear Mr./Madam Prime Minister:
Premier	His/Her Excellency (full name), Premier of _____	Excellency Dear Mr./Madam Premier:
President of a Republic	His/Her Excellency (full name)	Excellency Dear Mr./Madame President:
Secretary General of the United Nations	His/Her Excellency (full name) Secretary General of the United Nations	Dear Mr./Madam Secretary General:

State and local officials

Governor	The Honorable (full name) Governor of _____	Dear Governor (surname):
Lieutenant Governor	The Honorable (full name) Lieutenant Governor of _____	Dear Mr./Mrs./Ms.(surname):
Secretary of State	The Honorable (full name) Secretary of State of _____	Dear Mr./Madam Secretary:

Chief Justice of the
    State Supreme Court
	The Honorable (full name)
	Chief Justice, Supreme Court of
	    the State of _____
		Dear Mr./Madam Chief Justice:

State Senator	The Honorable (full name) The Senate of _____	Dear Senator (surname):
State Representative	The Honorable (full name) House of Representatives	Dear Mr./Mrs./Ms. (surname):
State Treasurer	The Honorable (full name) Treasurer of (state)	Dear Mr./Mrs./Ms. (surname):
Local Judge	The Honorable (full name) Judge of the Court of _____	Dear Judge (surname):
Mayor	The Honorable (full name) Mayor of _____	Dear Mayor (surname):
City Attorney	The Honorable (full name) (title) for the City of _____	Dear Mr./Mrs./Ms. (surname):
Commissioner	The Honorable (full name) Commissioner of _____	Dear Commissioner (surname):
Councilperson	The Honorable (full name) Councilman/Councilwoman	Dear Mr./Mrs./Ms.(surname):

Academic officials and professionals

President of a university or college	President (full name)	Dear Dr. (surname):
President who is a priest	The Very Reverend (full name)	Dear Father (surname):
Chancellor of a university	Dr./Mr./Mrs./Ms. (full name)	Dear Dr./Mr./Mrs./Ms. (surname):
Dean of a school, univer- sity or college	Dean (full name)	Dear Dean (surname):
Professor (with doctorate)	Dr. (full name) Professor of _____	Dear Dr. (surname):
Professor or instructor with no doctorate	Mr./Mrs./Ms. (full name)	Dear Mr./Mrs./Ms.(surname):
Attorney	Mr./Mrs./Ms. (full name) Attorney at Law	Dear Mr./Mrs./Ms.(surname):
Physician or surgeon	(full name), M.D. or Dr. (full name)	Dear Dr. (surname):
Dentist	(full name), D.D.S. or Dr. (full name)	Dear Dr. (surname):

Position or Title	Styling for Address	Styling for Salutation
Veterinarian	(full name), D.VM. or Dr. (full name)	Dear Dr. (surname):
Certified public accountant	(full name), C.P.A.	Dear Mr./Mrs./Ms.(surname):
Engineer or scientist with doctorate	Dr. (full name), (title)	Dear Dr. (surname):

Members of the clergy

Pope	His Holiness the Pope	Your Holiness:
Archbishop	The Most Reverence (full name) Archbishop of _____	Dear Archbishop (surname): My Dear Archdeacon:
Archdeacon	The Venerable (full name) Archdeacon of _____	
Cardinal	His Eminence Cardinal (full name)	Your Eminence:
Bishop, Roman Catholic	The Most Reverend (full name)	Dear Bishop (surname):
Bishop, Episcopal	The Right Reverend (full name)	Dear Bishop (surname):
Bishop, other denominations	The Reverend (full name) Bishop of _____	Dear Bishop (surname):
Dean of a cathedral	The Very Reverend (full name) Dean of _____	Dear Dean (surname):
Priest	The Reverend (full name)	Dear Father (surname):
Minister or pastor	The Reverend (full name)	Dear Reverend (surname):
Rabbi	Rabbi (full name)	Dear Rabbi (surname):
Mother Superior	The Reverend Mother Superior Convent of _____	Reverend Mother:
Sister, Roman Catholic	Sister (full name), (order)	Dear Sister (full name):
Military chaplain	Chaplain (full name) (rank and service)	Dear Chaplain (surname):

Military ranks

General*	General (full name) (branch of service)	Dear General (surname): .
Admiral*	Admiral (full name) (branch of service)	Dear Admiral (surname):
Colonel	Colonel (full name) (branch of service)	Dear Colonel (surname):
Major	Major (full name) (branch of service)	Dear Major (surname):

Position or Title	**Styling for Address**	**Styling for Salutation**
Captain	Captain (full name) (branch of service)	Dear Captain (surname):
Commander	Commander (full name) (branch of service)	Dear Commander (surname):

*It is common practice to show the specific rank, such as Major General; Lieutenant General; Rear Admiral; Vice Admiral; First Lieutenant; Lieutenant, i.g., if that rank is known to the sender. This distinction, however, is not made in the salutation.

Lieutenant*	Lieutenant (full name) (branch of service)	Dear Lieutenant (surname):
Chief Warrant Officer	Chief Warrant Officer (full name) (branch of service)	Dear Mr./Ms. (surname):
Petty Officer	Petty Officer (full name) (branch of service)	Dear Mr./Ms. (surname):
Ensign	Ensign (full name) (branch of service)	Dear Ensign (surname):
Master Sergeant	Master Sergeant (full name) (branch of service)	Dear Sergeant (surname):
Cadet	Cadet (full name) (branch of service)	Dear Cadet (surname):
Midshipman	Midshipman (full name) (branch of service)	Dear Midshipman (surname):

Appendix F:
Use of a Thesaurus

A thesaurus is a reference book containing synonyms—words having the same or nearly the same meaning as another word—and antonyms—words meaning the opposite of another word. Words are listed alphabetically like a dictionary. The purpose of a thesaurus is to vary the expressions of the entry word in order to provide more interesting writing. The best-known thesaurus is *Roget's*.

As an example, consider the entry for *medicine/medication*:

(N) Substance that helps cure, alleviate or prevent illness.

anesthetic, antibiotic, antidote, antiseptic, antitoxin, balm, biologic, capsule, cure, dose, drug, elixir, injection, inoculation, liniment, lotion, medicament, ointment, pharmaceutical, physic, pill, potion, prescription, remedy, salve, sedative, serum, tablet, tincture, tonic, vaccination, vaccine

Appendix G:
Use of the English Dictionary

A dictionary is a reference or resource book that contains a great deal of information, depending on its size and organization. The most common purposes of a dictionary are to provide the definitions and correct pronunciation of words and to identify parts of speech. But a dictionary, medical or English, may contain much more information:

capitalization and punctuation rules (English)
meaning of frequently used foreign terms
history of words (etymology)
comparisons of adjectives and adverbs (English)
proofreaders' marks
cross-references
various tables and charts

signs and symbols
measurements
bibliographies
illustrations
footnotes
diseases (medical)
units of measurement (medical)
guide for writers (English)

Each word listed in the dictionary is referred to as an *entry* word, which is broken into syllables. The phonetic spelling of the word indicating its pronunciation is found in parenthesis after the entry. The part of speech is usually identified in italic print (Figure A-1).

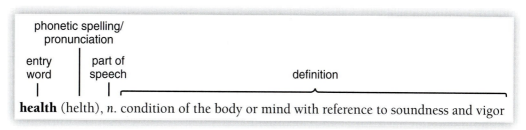

health (helth), *n.* condition of the body or mind with reference to soundness and vigor

FIGURE A-1 Dictionary word

To save time and facilitate the location of words in the dictionary, *guide words* are placed at the top of each page. The first guide word is the first word on the page. The second guide word is the last word on the page. All entries that fall *alphabetically* between the guide words are located on that page.

guide words: masthead ———————————————————————————— maw

Unfortunately, many words are spelled incorrectly because they are spoken incorrectly. That is why the respelling of words is so important. The respelling of the word *health* shows that the letter *a* is silent. On the other hand, the respelling of the word *khaki* shows that the phonetic respelling is quite different from the entry word.

health (helth)   khaki (kak'ē)

Note that the phonetic respelling uses symbols to assist in the pronunciation of words. To decipher the symbol, consult the pronunciation key found in every dictionary, whether at the bottom or side of each page, or in the front or back of the book. The accent mark after the first syllable (kak') shows which syllable to stress.

The most common phonetic symbols are the long and short vowels and the *schwa* that looks like an upside down letter *e* (ə). The schwa sounds like *uh* as in the word *about* (ə bout). The vowels are *a, e, i, o, u,* and sometimes *y.* Long vowels have the sound of their own letter name. The symbol above a long vowel is a short horizontal line (˘) called a *macron.*

Examples

ā ā, as in *late*   ī as in *ripe*   ū, as in *blue*

ē, as in *be*   ō, as in *note*

Short vowels have a small u-like symbol (˘) above the vowel called a *breve.*

Examples

ă ă, as in *bat*   ĭ, as in *it*   ŭ ŭ, as in *cut*

ĕ ĕ, as in *pet*   ŏ ŏ, as in *pot*

The symbols in the pronunciation key mean that the letters have the same sound as in vowels in these words:

ă ă, *pat*	oi, *boy*
ā, *pay*	ou, *cow*
âr, *car*	ŏo, *took*
âr, *father*	ŏo, *boot*
ā, *pet*	ŭ, *cut*
ē ĕ, *be*	ûr, *urge*
ĭ, *pit*	th, *thin, ether*

ī, *pie*

îr ir, *pier*

ō, *toe*

ô, *paw*

t, *attack, lateral*

hw, *which*

zh, *vision* \vi- ᶾ zs hen\

ə, *about* \ ə-bout\

Appendix H:
Use of the Medical Dictionary

A medical dictionary has most of the same features as an English dictionary—abbreviations, illustrations, tables, and symbols—but it focuses exclusively on medical terms and topics. Many medical entries have information beyond these features. For example, after the word *ostomy* is defined, further information is provided under subheadings titled ostomy care, stoma care, irrigation of colostomy, and miscellaneous considerations.

Other subheadings might include nursing implications, caution, nursing diagnoses, etiology, first aid, poisoning, prognosis, systems, and treatment. An appendix further augments medical information under the titles of anatomy, phobias, nutritional value of foods, minerals and vitamins, universal precautions, physical content of elements, dietary allowances, major diagnostic category (MDC), nursing diagnosis, medical emergencies, and diagnostic-related groups.

Entry words in the medical dictionary are not divided into syllables, nor do they provide the part of speech as found in the English dictionary. However, they do have phonetic spellings. Because medical words are long and difficult to pronounce, the respelling is especially helpful.

Examples

influenza (ĭn"floo-ĕn'-ză)

physiology (fĭz"ē-ŏl' ō-jē)

Glossary

Abstract nouns Nouns that name a concept, quality, or idea.

Action verbs Words that express activity rather than a state of being.

Active voice Indicates that the subject is doing, rather than receiving, the action.

Adjective A word that describes a noun or pronoun by giving more information about it

Adverb A word that describes or modifies a verb, adjective, or other adverb.

American Association of Medical Assistants (AAMA) The organization responsible for certification of individuals who have completed an accredited Medical-Assisting education and training program in the United States.

American Health Information Management Association (AHIMA) The leading organization in governing health information management, AHIMA promotes the best practices and standards fot the health information management community.

American Psychological Association (APA) style A style of scientific writing that was developed by behavioral and social scientists to standardize writing styles.

Antecedent The noun that a pronoun replaces; the antecedent usually appears before the pronoun.

Appositive A word or group of words that immediately follows and further identifies another noun.

Being verbs Verbs that express a state of being. Any form of the verb *to be* that stands alone (am, is, are, was, were, any form of be or been) is a being verb.

Chart notes, nurses notes, progress notes A description detailing the encounter specifics of a connection with a patient.

Clause A group of words that contains a subject and a verb.

Collective nouns Nouns that represent a group.

Comma splice An error that occurs when two or more independent clauses are incorrectly connected by a comma.

Common nouns Nouns that do not name any specific or particular person, place, object, or quality.

Comparative adjective An adjective that compares two persons, places, things, or ideas.

Comparative degree adverb An adverb that is used to compare two persons or things that perform the same action.

Complex sentence A sentence that contains one independent clause and one or more dependent clauses.

Compound adjectives Adjectives that combine two or more describing words that act as a single describer.

Compound prepositions Groups of two or three words that are used so frequently together that they function like one-word prepositions.

Compound sentence A sentence that contains two or more independent clauses but no dependent clause.

Compound subject A compound subject (two or more words joined by *and*) requires a plural verb.

Compound-complex sentence A sentence that contains two or more independent clauses and one or more dependent clauses.

Conciseness Expressing a lot of information in a few words; sentences are not cluttered with unnecessary words.

Concrete nouns Nouns that name things that are touchable, visible, and audible; that is, they are perceived by the senses.

Conjunction A word (*and, but, or, yet*) that joins words or parts of sentences. There are three types of conjunctions: coordinating, correlative, and subordinating.

Consultation report A report prepared for the referring physician when a consultation has been requested to obtain a second opinion on a problem or diagnosis; it contains the consulted physician's impressions, recommendations, evaluations, diagnoses, and treatment, as well as the results of any diagnostic procedures performed as part of the consultation.

Coordinating conjunctions Conjunctions (*and, but, or,* and *yet*) that are used to join two single words or groups of words of the same kind or of equal construction.

Correlative conjunctions Conjunctions that consist of two elements used as pairs to connect parallel structures.

Declarative sentence A sentence that makes known (declares) some type of information or statement. It ends with a period.

Degrees of adjectives Three degrees of comparison—positive, comparative, and superlative—that help describe the quality of a person, place, thing, or idea in comparison to another person, place, thing, or idea.

Degrees of adverbs Adverbs have three degrees of comparison: positive, comparative, and superlative.

Demonstrative pronouns Pronouns (*this, that, these,* and *those*) that point out people or

things at varying degrees of distance in space or time.

Dependent clause A clause that cannot stand alone. It always begins with a subordinating conjunction or a relative pronoun. Although it can contain a subject and a verb, it does not express a complete thought.

Descriptive adjectives Adjectives that modify nouns or pronouns by describing their characteristics or qualities.

Descriptive paragraph A pictorial representation in words that appears in most types of writing.

Diction The writer's choice of words and how those words are used in writing.

Direct address A noun, inserted into a message, that names the listener and makes the message more direct and personal.

Discharge summary A summary of the patient's condition during his or her stay at the facility.

Double negatives A grammatical error in Standard English; formed by using two negative words consecutively.

ECG (Electrocardiogram) A graphic record, or tracing, of the heart's electrical activity; produced by electrocardiography.

Empirical studies Research gaining knowledge by direct or indirect observation or analyzed quantitatively or qualitatively.

Eponyms Proper nouns or adjectives that name something derived from, and identified with, a real or mythical person.

Exclamatory sentences Sentences that express strong emotions. They end with an exclamation point.

Expository paragraph The most common type of paragraph; its purpose is to inform, explain, or define something.

Facsimile (FAX) Transmissions sent over telephone lines. Commonly used to send reports and documents in the medical care setting.

Finalizing stage The fourth step of the writing process, in which the final version is rewritten or retyped after all of the necessary corrections have been made to the writer's satisfaction.

Fragmented sentences Sentences that do not express a complete thought; some necessary information is omitted.

Full block letter A style of letter writing in which all lines are flush with the left margin.

Future tense Expresses action that will take place any time after the present time.

Gerund A verb form that ends in *-ing* and acts as a noun. It can be used in any way that a noun may be used.

Health Insurance Portability and Accountability Act of 1996 (HIPAA) Legislation that provides data privacy and security provisions for safeguarding medical information.

Helping verb A verb that is used together with a main verb to help express tense, mood, and voice.

History and Physical (H&P) report A collection of data about past events in relation to a patient's present illness. Usually dictated after a new patient is admitted to a hospital or comes to a clinic, office, or health facility.

Imperative sentences Sentences that give a command or make a request. They end with a period.

Indefinite articles *A* and *an* are limiting adjectives called indefinite articles.

Indefinite pronouns Pronouns that refer to persons or things in general.

Independent clause Called the main clause, it expresses a complete thought. An independent clause can stand alone as a sentence.

Infinitive A verb form that consists of the word *to* plus a verb; an infinitive usually acts as a noun.

Interrogative adjectives Adjectives that ask direct or indirect questions.

Interrogative pronouns Pronouns that are used simply to ask questions.

Interrogative sentences Sentences that ask direct questions. They end with a question mark.

Intransitive verbs Verbs that do not have a direct object to receive the action.

Joint Commission An organization responsible for accreditation of health care organizations and institutions, both in the United States and around the world.

Limiting adjective An adjective that limits the nouns to a definite or indefinite amount.

Linking verb A verb that connects the subject with a complement—a noun, pronoun, adjective, or phrase—that completes the meaning of the verb.

Manuscript Literally "written by hand," the manuscript is the document containing the processed copy—either handwritten or typed—of the writer's work.

Medical record A conglomeration and accumulation of data that documents and describes the history of a person's health care. Also known as Medical Charts, Health Records, Electronic Health Records, and Electronic Medical Records (EMR).

Methodology A body of methods, rules, or a set of ideas that are important to a science or art; a particular procedure or set of procedures.

Minutes The official (and sometimes legal) summary record of events and decisions that occur during a meeting.

Modified Block (Standard) letter A style of letter writing in which all of the lines are at the left margin except for the date and complimentary closing with signature.

Narrative paragraph A type of paragraph that tells a story or shows a series of events that usually occur in chronological order.

Negative adverbs Words that express a denial or a refusal; *no*, *not*, *never*, *nowhere*, *none*, *hardly*, *rarely*, *barely*, *scarcely*, and *seldom*.

Nominative case Nominative case refers to the subject of the verb in a sentence.

Noun A word that names a person, place, thing, or idea.

Object of a preposition A noun that follows a preposition.

Objective case: direct object A noun that follows a verb and names the person, place, thing, or idea that receives the action.

Objective case: indirect object A noun that follows a verb and names the person, place, or thing to whom, for whom, to what, or for what something was done.

Operative report A comprehensive description of a surgical procedure performed on a patient.

Paragraph A group of sentences that are related and explain a common point of view, or main idea, that the writer wishes to convey to the reader.

Parallel sentence structure Sentence structure in which words, phrases, and clauses are expressed in the same grammatical construction.

Participial phrase A word group consisting of a past participle (verb ending in -en) or a present participle (verb ending in -ing), plus any modifiers, objects, and complements. A participial phrase functions as an adjective and is used to modify a noun.

Past tense Expresses action that was completed in the past.

Pathology report A report that contains a description of tissue samples removed from the body for examination and diagnosis.

Personal pronouns Pronouns that refer to specific people and things.

Persuasive paragraph A paragraph that is written to urge the reader to follow a certain course of action, to deal with an important issue, or to state an opinion about a debatable issue.

Phrase A group of words without a subject combined with a verb.

Positive degree The base form of an adjective; describes nouns without making a comparison.

Positive degree adverb The base form of the adverb.

Possessive case Indicates possession or ownership. Formed by adding an apostrophe (') and an "s" to the appropriate noun or by using the appropriate possessive pronoun.

Predicate adjective An adjective that comes after linking verbs.

Predicate noun A noun that follows a linking verb and functions as another name for the subject.

Predicate noun A noun that follows a linking verb in a sentence and functions as another name for the subject.

Preposition A word that shows how a noun or pronoun is related to another word or a group of words

Prepositional noun/pronoun modifier A prepositional phrase that is used to modify a noun or pronoun in a sentence.

Prepositional phrase A group of words that begins with a preposition and ends with a noun or pronoun that is its object.

Prepositional verb modifiers Prepositional phrases that modify verbs and answer the questions *how? when? where?* and *to what extent?*

Present tense Expresses action that is happening at the present time, or action that happens regularly.

Prewriting stage The planning stage of the writing process, during which the author prepares an outline of everything he or she wants to write about the topic.

Problem-oriented medical record (POMR) A method of organizing a patient's record by charting the patient's problems in order of importance, as well as how those problems are addressed.

Promotional writing The type of writing that includes advertisements, press releases, announcements, brochures, and informational materials.

Pronoun A word that replaces or substitutes for a noun.

Proofreading stage The fifth and final stage of the writing process, the purpose of the proofreading stage is to check and correct the final printed product.

Proper adjective An adjective that has its source in a proper noun. Begins with a capital letter.

Proper noun A word that names a particular person, place, object, or quality.

Protected Health Information (PHI) Health information that is individually identifiable that is held or transmitted by a covered entity or its business associate, in any form or medium, whether electronic, on paper, or oral.

Punctuation A system of symbols used to make the written message easier to read and understand.

Radiology and imaging report A report that describes the results of a diagnostic procedure performed using radio waves or other forms of radiation.

Reflexive pronouns Pronouns that refer back to a noun or pronoun that appears earlier in the sentence.

Relative pronouns Pronouns that relate one part of a sentence to a word in another part of the sentence.

Research The activity of obtaining information about a subject. It involves such skills as planning, critical thinking, reading studies, and interviews.

Resume A summary of a person's job experience, education, and background skills; used as a reference by employers when interviewing a prospective employee.

Rewriting stage The third step of the writing process, in which the manuscript is reviewed and refined.

Run-on sentence An error that occurs when two or more independent clauses are joined together without punctuation.

Semi-Modified Block (Indented) letter A style of letter writing in which the first line of every paragraph is indented five spaces.

Sentence A group of words that expresses a complete thought.

Simple sentence A sentence formed with one independent clause and no dependent clause.

Simplified letter There is no salutation of complimentary closure with this style. All the lines are flush to the left margin.

Source-oriented medical record (SOMR) Patient data/information written in separate sections by health providers: nurses, doctors, medical assistants, labs.

Subjective-Objective-Assessment-Plan (SOAP) Part 4 of the POMR, these are progress notes that record a patient's description of his or her problems (Subjective), what the doctor, nurse, or medical assistant observes (Objective), assessments by the physician/provider (Assessment), and a treatment plan or medical interventions for the patient's medical problems (Plan).

Subordinating conjunction A conjunction that begins an adverb clause and joins the clause to the sentence.

Superlative adjective An adjective that compares three or more persons, places, things, or ideas.

Superlative degree adverb An adverb that is used to compare more than two persons or things that perform the same action.

The Department of Health and Human Services (DHHS) A department of the U.S. federal government; its goal is to protect the health of all Americans and to provide essential human services.

The Health Information Technology for Economic and Clinical Health Act of 2009 (HITECH) Legislation created to stimulate the adoption of the electronic health record (EHR).

The writing process The five steps of prewriting, writing, rewriting, finalizing, and proofreading that apply to any type of writing.

Transitive verb A verb that shows action and needs a direct object to complete its meaning.

Verb A word that shows action or a state of being.

Verb tenses Verb tenses specify the time—past, present, or future—of the action or state expressed by the verb.

Voices of verbs Show whether the subject of the verb is doing the action (active) or receiving the action (passive).

Writing stage The second step of the writing process, in which pencil is applied to paper or fingers to keyboard. The idea is to just write without worrying about spelling, grammar, or punctuation. Let anything happen.

Index

A

A and An, 88–89
AAMRL. *See* American Association of Medical Records Librarians (AAMRL)
Abbreviations
  in medical record, 78
  rules for, 135
Abstract noun, 6–7
Accreditation status, medical records and, 78
Action verb, 57–58
Active voice, 72–73
Addressing, of envelope, 28–29
Adjectives, 87–101
  as adverbs, 118–119
  clauses, 137–138
  commas between, 170
  degrees of, to express comparison
    comparative, 96–97
    positive, 96
    superlative, 97–98
  eponyms, 100–101
  modifiers and placement, 94–96
  placement of, 94
  as prepositional phrase, 139
  summary, 100
  troublesome, 99
  types
    descriptive, 92–93
    interrogative and proper, 90
  limiting, 88–89
  predicate and compound, 90–92
  singular and plural, 89
Adverbs, 113–122
  adjectives as, 118–119
  clauses, 138
  comparative, 116–117
  comparison, degrees to express, 116–118
  frequency, 116
  irregular, 117–118
  as modifiers, 115–116
  negative, 119–121
  placement of, 121
  positive, 116
  as prepositional phrase, 139
  recognizing, 113–115
  summary, 122
  superlative, 117
  troublesome, 121–122
Advertisement, 215–217
AHIMA. *See* American Health Information Management Association (AHIMA)
American Association of Medical Records Librarians (AAMRL), 77
American College of Surgeons, 77
American Health Information Management Association (AHIMA), 77
American Medical Record Association (AMRA), 77
AMRA. *See* American Medical Record Association (AMRA)
An and A, 88–89

Antecedent, pronoun agreement with, 45–46
APA (American Psychological Association), 214–218
Apostrophe
    with possessive case, 12–13
    punctuation, 178
Appositives, 14–15, 171
Appropriate wording, guidelines for, 231–232
Arabic numbers, rules for, 257–258
ARLNA. *See* Association of Record Librarians of North
        America (ARLNA)
Association of Record Librarians of North America
        (ARLNA), 77

B

Being verb, 58
Blind carbon copy (BCC), 51
Block style letter, 18–19
Body, of medical letter, 24–25
Brand names, 5
Brochures, 215–217

C

Can and may, 70–71
Capitalization, rules for, 255–256
Carbon copy (CC), 51
Cases
    nouns
        nominative, 10
        objective, 11–12
        possessive case, 12–13
    of personal pronouns, 37–40
Cause and effect, paragraph organization, 210
Charting, 157–162
    PIE method, 160–161
    SOAP method, 158–159
    SOAPE method, 160
    SOAPIE method, 160
    SOAPIER method, 160
    summary, 161–162
    traditional, 158
Chronological resume, 243–244
Classification paragraph organization, 211
Clauses
    adjective, 137–138
    adverb, 138
    dependent, 136–138
    independent, 136–138
    independent clauses, 170
    nouns as, 137

Clichés, rules for, 259–260
Clinical record, 76–77
Closing, of medical letter, 24–27
Collective noun, 5–6
Colon, 175–176
Combination/hybrid resume, 244–246
Comma, 170–173
Comma splice, 153
Common name, 4
Common noun, 4–5
Comparative adjectives, 96–97
Comparative adverbs, 116
Comparative degree of comparison, 96–97
Comparisons
    degrees of adjectives to express, 96–99
    degrees of adverbs to express, 116–118
    paragraph organization by, 210–211
Complex sentences, 142
Components of sentences, 136–141
Compound adjectives, 90–92
Compound prepositions, 193–194
Compound sentences, 141–142
Compound-complex sentences, 142
Computer writing, guidelines for, 234
Conciseness
    effective sentences, 146–149
    in writing, 232
Concluding sentence, in paragraph, 207
Concrete noun, 6
Confidentiality, of medical records, 79–81
Conjunctions, 200–202
Consonants, doubling rule for, 252–253
Consultation reports, 185–186
Contractions, not as, 119–120
Coordinating conjunctions, 200
Correct grammar, in writing, 233
Correlative conjunctions, 200
Cover letter, 246–248

D

Dash, 177
Data base, 158
Dates, commas in, 170–171
Declarative sentences, 143
Deduction, paragraph organization by, 210
Definition, paragraph organization by, 211
Demonstrative pronouns, 44
Dependent clause, 136–138
Dependent clauses, 136–138
Descriptive adjectives, 92–93

Descriptive paragraph, 205–206
Diction, in effective sentences, 149–150
Dictionary
    medical dictionary, 270
    use of English, 267–269
Direct address, nouns and, 14–15
Direct object, noun, 11–12
Discharge summary, 104–105
Documentation, in medical records, 78
Double comparison, 98
Double negatives, 120

E

Effective sentences
    conciseness, 146–149
    diction, 149–150
    parallel structure, 145
    positive statement, 151
Ei/ie spelling rule, 251
Electronic mail, 48–53
Electronic Medical Records (EMR), 77
EMR. *See* Electronic Medical Records (EMR)
English dictionary, 267–269
Eponyms, 5, 100–101
Exclamation point, 169
Exclamatory sentences, 144
Explicitness, in writing, 232
Expository paragraph, 206

F

Facsimile, 123–124
Feminine pronoun, 36
Finalizing, 230
Fragmented sentences, 152
Frequency adverbs, 116
Full block style, 18–19
Functional resume, 243–245
Future tense verbs, 64

G

Gender
    in pronoun, 36
    pronoun-antecedent agreement, 45–46
Generic names, 5
Gerunds, 61, 140
Grammar
    correctness in writing, 233
    defined, 3

H

Heading, of medical letter, 18, 22
Headings, of manuscripts, 215
Health Insurance Portability and Accountability Act (HIPAA), 77, 79–81
Helping verbs, 59
HIPAA laws. *See* Health Insurance Portability and Accountability Act (HIPAA)
History and physical medical reports, 183–186
Hybrid/combination resume, 244–246
Hyphen, 177–178

I

Imperative mood, 74
Imperative sentences, 143
Inclusive language, in writing style, 233
Indefinite pronouns, 42–43
Indented style, 18, 21
Independent clauses, 136–138, 170
Indicative mood, 74
Indirect object
    noun, 11
    pronoun, 39
Induction, paragraph organization by, 210
Ineffective sentences
    comma splice, 153
    fragmented, 152
    run-on, 153–154
Infinitives, 61, 140–141
Information sheets, 217–218
Initial plan, 158
Inside address, of medical letter, 21, 23
Interoffice memorandum, 48–53
Interrogative adjectives, 90
Interrogative pronouns, 43
Interrogative sentences, 143
Intransitive verbs, 60–61
Irregular adjectives, 99
Irregular adverbs, 117–118
Irregular verbs, 66–68
Italics, 179
Its and It's, use of, 46

J

JCAHO. *See* Joint Commission on Accreditation of Healthcare Organizations (JCAHO)
Joint Commission on Accreditation of Healthcare Organizations (JCAHO), 78

K

Keywords for resumes, 242–243

L

Legibility, of medical records, 78
Lie and lay, 69
Limiting adjectives, 88–89
Linking verbs
  defined, 59–60
  predicate nouns and, 10–11
  prepositional modifiers, 196–197
Litigation, medical records in, 78
Location, paragraph organization
      and, 210

M

Main verb, 59
Manuscript
  defined, 214
  preparation guidelines
    APA writing style, 214–215
    format guidelines, 214–218
    headings, 215
Masculine noun, 4–5
Masculine pronoun, 36
May and can, 70–71
Medical chart, 77. *see also* Charting
Medical dictionary, 270
Medical office correspondence
  addressing envelopes for, 28–29
  electronic mail, 48–53
  envelopes for, 28–29
  facsimile, 123–124
  interoffice memorandum, 48–53
  medical letter
    body, 24–25
    closing and signature, 24–27
    folding, 29
    formats and presentation, 17–18
    heading, 18, 22
    inside address, 21, 23
    meeting minutes, 125–126
    notations, 25–27
    phone messages, 123–125
    salutation, 23
    styles of, 17–22
    subject line, 24
  Medical record

documentation rules, 78
  essential information in, 76–77
  features of, 78
  language of, 76–81
  legal uses for, 78
  privacy and confidentiality issues, 79–81
  problem-oriented medical record (POMR)
      method, 158
  standards for, 77–78
Medical reports
  consultation reports, 185–186
  discharge summary, 104–105
  history and physical reports, 183–186
  operative report, 104, 106
  pathology report, 103–104
  punctuation, 167–186
  radiology and imaging reports, 102–103
Medical spelling lists, 17, 48, 76, 101, 122, 157, 183,
      203, 214, 235
Medical terms, plurals in, 7–9
Meeting minutes, 125–126
Memorandum, office, 48–53
Minutes, of meetings, 125–126
Misplaced modifiers, 94–96
Modified block style (standard), 18, 20
Modifiers
  adverbs as, 115–116
  placement of adjectives, 94–96
  prepositional noun/pronoun modifiers, 195
  prepositional verb modifiers, 196–197
Moods, of verbs, 74

N

Narrative paragraph, 205
Negative adverbs, 119–121
Neuter pronouns, 36
Nominative case
  in personal pronoun, 37–38
  subject, 10
Not, as contraction, 119–120
Nouns, 3–18
  characteristics and functions
      functions, 9–15
      number, 7–9
  clauses, 137
  clauses and phrases, 137
  modifiers, 114
  prepositional modifiers, 195
  in prepositional phrases, 195–197
  prepositional phrases as, 139

summary, 15–16
types
abstract, 6–7
collective, 5–6
common, 4–5
concrete, 6
proper, 4–5
Number
in noun, 7–9
in pronoun, 36–37
pronoun-antecedent agreement, 45
usage rules for, 257–258
of verb, 62–63

O

Object of preposition, 11–12
Object pronoun, 39
Objective case
in noun, 11–12
in personal pronoun, 39
Office memorandum
structure of, 48–52
writing guidelines for, 48–53
Operative report, 104, 106
Organization, of medical records, 78

P

Paragraph, 203–213
cause and effect organization, 210
comparison organization, 210–211
deductive organization, 210
definition or classification organization, 211
definition-based organization, 211
descriptive, 205–206
examples of, 203–204
expository, 206
inductive organization, 210
location organization, 210
narrative, 205
organization, 209–211
persuasive, 206–207
structure of, 207–209
concluding sentence, 207
supporting sentences, 207
topic sentence, 207
summary, 213
time organization, 209–210
types of, 205–207
unity, 212–213

Parallel structure, effective sentences, 145
Parentheses, 176–177
Parenthetical expressions, punctuation of, 172
Participial phrase, 139–140
Parts of speech, 3–4
Passive verbs, 72–73
Passive voice, identification of, 72–73
Past participles, 65
Past tense, 63–64
Pathology report, 103–104
Period, 168–169
Person, of verb, 61–62
Personal pronouns
gender, 36
nominative case, 37–38
number and person, 36–37
objective case, 39
possessive case, 39–40
pronoun-antecedent agreement, 45–46
Persuasive paragraph, 206–207
Phone messages, 123–125
Phrases, 138–141
commas, 171–172
prepositional, 139
summary, 155–157
verbal
gerund, 140
infinitive, 140–141
participial, 139–140
Physician's Desk Reference (PDR), 5
Plurals
adjectives as, 89
medical terms, 7–9
in nouns, 7–9
POMR. *See* Problem-oriented medical record (POMR)
method
Positive adverbs, 116
Positive degree of comparison, 96
Positive statements, in effective sentences, 151
Possessive case, 12–13, 39–40
Possessive nouns, 12–13
Predicate adjectives, 90–92
Predicate noun, 10–11
Predicate pronouns, 38
Prepositional phrases, 139, 195–197
Prepositions
compound prepositions, 193–194
defined, 191–193
at end of sentence, 199–200
noun/pronoun modifiers, 195
object of, 11–12

Prepositions (*Continued*)
  problematic, 197–199
  summary, 201–202
  verb modifiers, 196–197
Present participles, verbs, 65
Present tense, 63
Prewriting, 228
Privacy, of medical records, 79–81
Problem lists, 158
Problematic prepositions, 197–199
Problem-Intervention-Evaluation (PIE) charting,
    160–161
Problem-oriented medical record (POMR)
    method, 158
Progress notes, 158
Promotional writing
  information sheets, 217–218
  sample brochure, 215–217
Pronouns, 36–47
  antecedent agreement with
    gender, 45–46
    number, 45
    person, 47
  defined, 35
  prepositional modifiers, 195
  in prepositional phrases, 195–197
  summary, 47
  types of
    demonstrative, 44
    indefinite, 42–43
    interrogative, 43
    personal, 36–40
    reflexive, 40–41
    relative, 41–42
  usage forms, 47
Proofreading, 230
Proper adjectives, 90
Proper noun, 4–5
Publication Manual of the American Psychological
    Association, 214
Punctuation, 167–182
  apostrophe, 178
  colon, 175–176
  comma, 170–173
  dash, 177
  exclamation point, 169
  hyphen, 177–178
  italics, 179
  parentheses, 176–177
  period, 168–169
  question mark, 169

  quotation marks, 180
  semicolon, 173–174
  summary, 181–182
Purpose, of writing, 231

Q

Question marks, 169
Quotation marks, 180

R

Radiology and imaging reports, 102–103
Raise and rise, 69–70
Reflexive pronouns, 40–41
Regular verbs, 65–66
Relative pronouns, 41–42
Report, defined, 214
Research paper
  defined, 214
  writing guidelines, 214–218
Resumes, 241–246
  completing, 245
  essentials of, 241–242
  keywords for, 242–243
  objective of, 242
  types of, 243–245
Rewriting, 229–230
Rise and raise, 69–70
Roman numerals, rules for, 257–258
Run-on sentences, 153–154

S

Salutations
  in medical letter, 23
  punctuations of, 172
  rules for, 261–265
Semicolon, 173–174
Semi-modified block (indented) style, 18, 21
Sentences
  adjectives in, 87–88
  classifications, 143–144
  comma splice, 153
  complex, 142
  components of, 136–141
  compound, 141–142
  compound-complex, 142
  concluding, 207
  declarative, 143
  dependent clauses, 136–138

effective
 conciseness, 146–149
 diction, 149–150
 parallel structure, 145
 positive statement, 151
exclamatory, 144
imperative, 143
independent clauses, 136–138
ineffective
 comma splice, 153
 fragmented, 152
 run-on sentence, 153–154
interrogative, 143
nouns in, 3–4
paragraph structure and, 207
prepositions at end of, 199–200
run-on, 153–154
simple, 141
structure, 141–142
summary, 155–157
supporting sentence, 207
topic sentence, 207
verb tenses in, 72
Signature
 on medical letter, 24–27
 in medical record, 78
Silent e, spelling rules, 253
Simple sentence, 141
Simple tense, 68
Simplified style, 18, 22
Singular adjectives, 89
Singular nouns, 7–9
Smoothness, in writing style, 233
SOAP (subjective-objective-assessment plan) charting
 method, 158–159
SOAPE charting method, 160
SOAPIE charting method, 160
SOAPIER charting method, 160
Spelling rules, 251–254
 consonant doubling, 252–253
 ei or ie, 251
 medical spelling, 17, 48, 76, 101, 122, 157, 183, 203,
  214, 235
 silent e, 253
 suffixes with y and c, 254
Standard style, 18, 20
Subject, nominative case, 10
Subject line, of medical letter, 24
Subjective-objective-assessment plan (SOAP) charting
 method, 158–159
Subjunctive mood, 74

Subordinating conjunctions, 201
Suffixes, y and c, spelling rules, 254
Superlative adjectives, 97–98
Superlative adverbs, 117
Supporting sentences, in paragraph, 207

T

Tenses, verbs, 63–65, 72
Thesaurus, use guidelines, 266
Time, paragraph organization and, 209–210
Timeliness, of medical records, 78
Titles (in salutations), rules for, 261–265
Topic sentence, in paragraph, 207
Trade names, 5
Traditional charting, 158
Transitive verb, 60–61
Troublesome adjectives, 99
Troublesome adverbs, 121–122

U

Unity, in paragraphs, 212–213

V

Verbal phrases
 gerund, 140
 infinitive, 140–141
 participial, 139–140
Verbs, 57–76
 modifiers, 114
 moods of, 74
 number of, 62–63
 person of, 61–62
 prepositional modifiers, 196–197
 principal parts
  confusing and troublesome verbs, 69–71
  irregular verbs, 66–68
  regular verbs, 65–66
 summary, 75–76
 tenses, 63–65, 72
 types of
  action, 57–58
  being, 58
  gerunds, 61
  helping, 59
  infinitives, 61
  intransitive, 60–61
  linking, 59–60
  main, 59

Verbs (*Continued*)
    transitive, 60–61
    voices of, 72–73

W

Weed, Lawrence, 158
Writing Guidelines
    cover letter, 246–247
    resumes
        completing of, 245
        essentials of, 241–242
        keywords for, 242–243
        objective of, 242
        types of, 243–245
Writing guidelines
    computer writing, 234
    electronic mail, 48–53
    manuscript preparation
        APA writing style, 214–218
        format guidelines, 214–218

office memos, 48–53
promotional writing, 216–218
writing process
    finalizing, 230
    prewriting, 228
    proofreading, 230
    rewriting, 229–230
    worksheets, 227
    writing, 228
writing style
    APA writing style, 214–218
    appropriateness, 231–232
    conciseness, 232
    correct grammar, 233
    explicitness, 232
    inclusive language, 233
    in medical record, 78
    purpose, 231
    smoothness, 233
    summary, 235